Systems Theory and the Sociology of Health and Illness

T0227587

Modern societies and organisations are characterised by multiple kinds of observations, systems, or rationalities, rather than singular identities and clear hierarchies. This holds true for health care where we find a range of different perspectives – from medicine to education, from science to law, from religion to politics – brought together in different types of arrangements. This innovative volume explores how this polycontexturality plays out in the health-care arena.

Drawing on systems theory, and Luhmann's theory of social systems as communicative systems in particular, the contributors investigate how things – drugs, for example – and bodies are observed and constructed in different ways under polycontextural conditions. They explore how the different types of communication and observation are brought into workable arrangements – without becoming identical or reconciled – and discuss how health-care organisations observe their own polycontexturality.

Providing an analysis of health-care structures that is up to speed with the complexity of health care today, this book shows how society and its organisations simultaneously manage contexts that do not fit together. It is an important work for those with an interest in health and illness, social theory, Niklas Luhmann, organisations and systems theory from a range of backgrounds including sociology, health studies, political science and management.

Morten Knudsen has been working with systems theory and health-care organisations for more than fifteen years. He has studied decision-making, the organisation of patient participation, standardisation and leadership development programmes within health-care organisations. He currently holds the position of Associate Professor in Organisational Analysis, Department of Organisation, Copenhagen Business School.

Werner Vogd is Professor and Chair of Sociology at Witten/Herdecke University, Germany. He has done work on medical decision-making processes in hospitals in the area of conflict between systems rationality and purposive rationality, as well as published a series of contributions to the fields of the sociology of organizations, medical sociology, sociological theory, systems theory, the sociology of religion, and the sociology of knowledge. He is currently managing a large empirical research-project on decision-making in contemporary German hospital management.

Routledge Studies in the Sociology of Health and Illness

Systems Theory and the Sociology of Health and Illness

Observing healthcare

Edited by Morten Knudsen and Werner Vogd

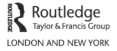

Routledge
Taylor & Francis Group

LONDON AND NEW YORK

First published 2015
by Routledge

2 Park Square, Milton Park, Abingdon OX14 4RN
and
711 Third Avenue, New York, NY 10017

First issued in paperback 2017

Routledge is an imprint of the Taylor & Francis Group, an informa business

British Library Cataloguing-in-Publication Data
A catalogue record for this book is available from the British Library

Library of Congress Cataloguing in Publication data
    Systems theory and the sociology of health and illness : observing
    healthcare / edited by Morten Knudsen and Werner Vogd.
        p. ; cm. – (Routledge studies in the sociology of health and illness)
    Includes bibliographical references and index.
    I. Knudsen, Morten, editor. II. Vogd, Werner, editor. III. Series: Routledge
    studies in the sociology of health and illness.
    [DNLM: 1. Delivery of Health Care. 2. Health Policy. 3. Social
    Medicine. 4. Systems Theory. W 84.1]
    RA418
    362.1–dc23
    2014019983

ISBN 13: 978-1-138-50340-3 (pbk)
ISBN 13: 978-1-138-79491-7 (hbk)

Typeset in Sabon
by Out of House Publishing

Contents

Illustrations

Figures

Tables

Contributors

Niels Åkerstrøm Andersen is Professor and Reseach Manager at the Department of Management, Politics and Philosophy, Copenhagen Business School, Denmark.

Jennifer Burr, Ph.D., is a senior lecturer in medical sociology at the School of Health and Related Research, University of Sheffield.

Barry J. Gibson, Ph.D., is a reader in medical sociology, Unit of Dental Public Health, School of Clinical Dentistry, University of Sheffield.

Anna Henkel, Ph.D., is an associate professor for social theory, Institute of Social Sciences, Carl von Ossietzky Universität Oldenburg.

Holger Højlund, Ph.D., is an associate professor at the Department of Management, Politics and Philosophy, at the Copenhagen Business School, Denmark.

Till Jansen, Ph.D., is a research assistant at the Chair for Leadership and Dynamics in Family Businesses at the University of Witten/Herdecke.

Hanne Knudsen, Ph.D., is an associate professor of educational management in the Department of Education, Aarhus University, Denmark.

Morten Knudsen, Ph.D., is an associate professor in organisational analysis in the Department of Organisation at the Copenhagen Business School.

Anders la Cour, Ph.D., is an associate professor at the Department of Management, Politics and Philosophy, at the Copenhagen Business School, Denmark.

Daniel Lüdecke is a senior researcher in the Department of Medical Sociology, University Medical Centre Hamburg-Eppendorf.

Katharina Mayr is a university lecturer in sociological theory, sociology of knowledge and professions at the Institute of Sociology, Ludwig Maximilian University Munich.

Dimitris Michailakis, Ph.D., is a professor of sociology and social welfare in the Department of Social and Welfare Studies, Linköping University, Sweden.

Armin Nassehi, Ph.D., is a professor in sociological theory, sociology of culture, political sociology, sociology of religion and sociology of knowledge at the Institute of Sociology, Ludwig Maximilian University Munich.

Sarah Poranzke is a Ph.D. student at the Chair for Sociology at the University of Witten/Herdecke.

Irmhild Saake, Ph.D., is a university lecturer in sociological theory, biographical research, thanatology and qualitative research at the Institute of Sociology, Ludwig Maximilian University Munich.

Werner Schirmer, Ph.D., is an associate professor in sociology in the Department of Social and Welfare Studies, University of Linköping, and a guest professor at the Centre for Social Theory, Ghent University.

Werner Vogd, Prof. Dr, is a professor in sociology at the Fakultät für Kulturreflexion, University Witten/Herdecke.

Acknowledgements

The editors would like to thank the Public-Private Platform at Copenhagen Business School for kindly sponsoring a workshop that discussed previous versions of the chapters in this book.

Introduction

Health care, systems theory and polycontexturality

Morten Knudsen and Werner Vogd

What is a patient? From a medical point of view, a patient is an ill or injured person (as defined by means of a diagnosis) under medical treatment or care; in a financial context, a patient is a cost (or an income); in a legal context, a patient is a subject with legal rights; for the mass media, patients represent a good story if their treatment does not match our expectations (that a hospital will help and not harm us, for instance). Thus, the relatively simple question of 'What is a patient?' is not so easy to answer. It turns out that the most general answer is, 'It depends on the observer.'

Not only patients but also doctors, nurses and managers, as well as risk and responsibility, are observed in multifarious ways. Today, a sundry range of means and ways of observation are involved in the development and organisation of health care, spanning from medicine to education, from science to law and religion to politics. Contemporary medical treatment is shaped by a set of specialised forms of observation, each of which comes with varying kinds of communication organised in assorted constellations with different types of complexity.

We are witnessing a current health-care situation in which differing and incommensurable types of observation and communication coexist with dependencies and mutual observations. This complex situation is the starting point of this book. Drawing on the latest sociological systems theory and with health care as the common empirical focus, the book investigates various aspects of the described multi-observer arrangements, or 'polycontexturality', as we shall call it. It explores how multiple types of communication and observation are brought into workable arrangements – without becoming identical or reconciled. The goal of the book is to provide descriptions that reflect the complexity of health care today. Health care is a particularly relevant empirical setting for a study of polycontexturality due to its complexity, which comprises multiple contextures such as medicine, economics, politics, law and science that form different arrangements. Health care is, as such, an extreme case of polycontexturality.

The analyses presented in the book draw on sociological systems theory, particularly the concepts of functional differentiation, polycontexturality and polyphony. This introduction presents these central concepts, relates them briefly to cognate concepts and then offers a concise presentation of the chapters of the book.

The theory of social systems

Sociological systems theory is the point of departure of this book, the works of Niklas Luhmann working as a common frame of reference (for introductions to Luhmann in English, see Borch 2011 and Moeller 2006, 2012). Luhmann's goal was to develop a new theory of society that could be used to analyse all social phenomena within a consistent conceptual frame. At the same time, Luhmann was quite eclectic in his choice of theories in that he incorporated and transformed concepts from different scientific branches, ranging from biology and philosophy to cybernetics and communication theory. From general systems theory, Luhmann inherited the idea of generating a type of theory universal enough to cover a variety of social areas, but one which could also be used and developed in analyses of specific empirical phenomena and their particularities. His theory is based on the assumption that areas such as economics, religion, medicine, science and education share basic similarities. Thus, 'systems theory' is a combination of general theories and theories of specific social systems and phenomena. In more than fifty books and roughly 500 journal articles, Luhmann developed a comprehensive and general theory of social systems (1995a), a theory of society (2012–13), several highly important function systems, organisations (2000a) and theories on more specific subjects such as risk (1993), trust and power (1979).

Within the sociology of health and illness, systems theory is typically associated with Parsons (Parsons 1979: 428 ff.; White 2009: 105 ff.). Of note, however, Luhmann developed a new and different theoretical perspective on how to observe modern society. Parsons assumed that social systems must have a shared value system and perform certain functions to be maintained. Luhmann, in contrast, did not wish to operate with pre-empirical structures. Social systems do not, he claims, need collectively shared values (Luhmann 1970: 113 ff.). Instead, he suggested an operatively defined concept of system, where a system consists of self-referential operations – and in so doing also makes a difference to the environment. A system can therefore also be defined as a difference, namely the difference between system and environment (Luhmann 1995a: 16 ff.). This means that Luhmann does not have to assume pre-given structures, identities or functions. He suggests a comparative functionalism that studies and compares different constellations of problems and solutions (Luhmann 1970, 1995a: 52 ff.; Knudsen 2010). This approach gives Luhmann's systems theory an unprecedented richness of themes, ideas and insights. Indicative of the theory's depth is the fact that three dictionaries covering the concepts developed by Luhmann have already been published (Krause 1996; Baraldi *et al.* 1997; Jahraus *et al.* 2012).

Even though Luhmann is increasingly acknowledged as one of the most important and original sociologists of the twentieth century, his work and ideas have seldom been applied to the sociology of health and illness. Luhmann himself only wrote a few minor pieces on medical issues (1983a, 1983b, 1990b; see also Stollberg 2009). This book argues that systems theory has something to offer the sociology of health and illness field. A broad area, sociology of health and illness has focused on the medical system (medical knowledge, professionals) and patients (their experience of illness, social inequalities) – and the interactions between them. The systems-theory focus on polycontexturality provides a different perspective as it centres on various aspects of the many contextures involved and how they are arranged. Systems theory has also been called the second-order observation theory because it observes observations. The object of study is not illness or the relationship between illness and living conditions, gender, race and the like. The object of study is communication: about illness, living conditions, gender, race and the like.

Functional differentiation

The theory of functional differentiation forms a cornerstone in Luhmann's theory of modern society. (For the most comprehensive presentation, see Luhmann 2013: 1–166.) Differentiation is a classical issue in sociology. Marx (1989) studied the differentiation between capital and work, while Simmel (1989) examined differentiation in relation to individualisation. Durkheim (1984) analysed it as the division of labour, and Weber looked at it as the emergence of different spheres of value and rationalities (Schimank 2007: 49 ff.). Differentiation is also a core theme for recent sociologists such as Habermas and Bourdieu, who use it in their theories of society, the former in his distinction between systems and life world (Habermas 1988) and the latter in his concept of different fields (Bourdieu 1998).

A new theory of differentiation is one of Luhmann's major sociological contributions. According to systems theory, society has various types of differentiation: segmentary (differentiated in equal systems), centre/periphery (typically as territorial inequality), stratificatory (differentiated in unequal subsystems based on ranks and status) and functional (based on societal function) (Luhmann 2013: 87 ff.). The various types of differentiation exist simultaneously, but functional differentiation has gained primacy today.

Functional differentiation means that society becomes differentiated in operationally closed, autonomous communicative systems. At present, society does not have a centre or a top but is characterised by the coexistence of different function systems, with different codes guiding their observations and giving them certain criteria of relevance. The most prominent function systems are law, economy, politics, art, education, science, religion, love, medicine and the mass media. They all observe their environments differently based on different codes and programmes. The tasks of one system cannot be taken over by another system. For instance, the legal system can stabilise normative expectation but not treat diseases; the medical system can treat diseases but not make collectively binding decisions; the political system can do that but not generate new knowledge. Function systems are not identical with organisations. Instead, the presence of function systems can be defined as what runs across the same type of organisations. The reason we recognise hospitals as hospitals, schools as schools, and courts as courts is that they relate to similar function systems (in this case, the medical, the pedagogical and the legal function system).

Historically, functional differentiation is a complicated process with many different preconditions. The central development is what could be called a codification of codes, which is the processes in which science, politics, law, medicine and other function systems begin to realise the recursivity of their own autopoietical reproduction (Luhmann 1997a: 708; Harste 2013). The timing and the processes differ between the different systems, and for centuries tensions existed between stratification and functional differentiation. Luhmann claims that since the end of the eighteenth century a more and more targeted distancing of functional systems from premises and the influence of classes has arisen (Luhmann 1980: 162 ff.). Legally, for example, the neutral legal subject is invented and the pedagogical system is oriented towards public schools for the entire population. Origin currently does not play a crucial role for the function systems. This does not exclude inequality in, for instance, health-care conditions or educational opportunities in relation to social background. But the medical system and its programmes do not distinguish between the rich and the poor body per se, and the pedagogical system does not give you better grades because your parents are rich.

Function systems evolve around a binary code that gives the system a criterion for whether its operations and programmes can connect or not (Vogd 2004: 117). The legal code is legal/illegal, meaning that every observation is filtered through this code. Everything that cannot obtain resonance in this code remains unobserved by the legal system. This means that the different function systems have a high degree of sensibility to specific issues but also a high degree of indifference towards everything else (Luhmann 1987: 57 ff.). The legal system is thus expected to concern itself with the law and be indifferent to the social status of the prosecuted. This expectation can be observed in the uproar if the legal system is perceived as systematically judging black people harder than white people. All men are created equal – is the expectation. Likewise, functional differentiation does not, of course, mean that no doctors have been influenced by pharmaceutical companies. The reason we find too tight relations between health care and the pharmaceutical industry highly problematic, however, must be seen based on the fact that we take functional differentiation for granted.

The codes of the different function systems are relatively stable but need further specification. The medical code of ill/well, for instance, is therefore supplemented by programmes that specify when something is defined as ill, what the disease is and how further communication should connect to the disease. Medical programmes do this, and there is a huge amount of rapidly changing medical programmes for making diagnoses and undertaking treatment, care and rehabilitation. The programmes can be and are revised, expanded and forgotten. The programmes specify the use of the code and structure the connecting communications. What is observed as disease is not given once and for all but changes with the medical programmes.

Like other functional systems, the medical system is operatively closed. This means that other systems cannot decide what should count as a disease and other systems cannot make programmes for diagnoses or treatments. The political system may of course try to influence the medical system (as the medical system may try to influence the political system), but it is the medical system that decides how it will react to such attempts. The medical system can let itself be informed by scientific results but is itself not a subsystem of the scientific system. Discussions on evidence-based medicine show that the medical system provides treatment even if the knowledge is uncertain, which it normally is as the situation is typically overly complex in relation to the knowledge available (Vogd 2005).

Functional differentiation should not be understood as a division of labour in the Durkheim sense, i.e. as unities specialised in specific tasks in the frames of a societal unit and with common benefits as a result (Borch 2011: 89). One could claim that Luhmann's analyses of function systems are closer to Foucault's analysis of the medical gaze (and later Foucault's notion of episteme) (2003). Function systems are specific perspectives on the world, specific observations that are different constructions of reality. Luhmann's theory of functional differentiation can be seen as a generalisation of the idea of a certain medical gaze, which is why we should also talk about, for instance, the economic, legal, scientific and religious gaze. Medical knowledge is not the only area that is constructed and has performative effects; this is also true for, for example, economic, legal and scientific knowledge.

Luhmann does not, however, talk about gazes; instead, a concept of observation becomes increasingly central in his theoretical architecture. According to systems theory, social systems consist of communication and nothing but communication. Communication is taken to be autopoietic or self-creating. Communication is the operation that constitutes social systems and can be studied in many different ways. In his later works, Luhmann studied communication increasingly as observations. Communication involves observation since it is communication about something that is thus also being observed (be it the weather, prices, a movie or my feelings).

Following the mathematician George Spencer Brown (1972), Luhmann defined observation as an indication in the context of a distinction (1998: 68 ff.). All observations depend on distinctions. For instance, the legal system can be characterised as communication that observes its environment from the standpoint of the distinction (i.e. code) between legal and illegal, while the scientific system observes from the perspective of the distinction true/false. Luhmann's book on ecological communication (1989), which illustrates this well, asks how society and its function systems can observe and react to environmental problems. The point is that society only responds to environmental problems in accordance with the codes and programmes that structure the observations of the societal systems. Which environmental problems are perceived as 'real' depends on *how* they are observed. The economic function system can only observe and react to disturbances that are expressed in the language of prices. Similarly the legal system, for instance, is only capable of resonance in accordance with its own structures, that is its code and programmes. Only environmental dangers that can be observed as either legal or illegal can be observed by the legal system.

Luhmann related to philosopher Gotthard Günther and his notions of contexture and polycontexturality in order to capture this epistemological perspective on functional differentiation. Because the purpose of this book is to explore various aspects of polycontexturality and how this concept can throw light on current issues in the sociology of health and illness, we shall unfold the concept further.

Polycontexturality

The concept of polycontexturality originated in the logic of Günther, who was heavily influenced by Hegel but also fascinated by cybernetics in the American context. Polycontexturality as defined by Günther is part of a philosophical logic with its own agenda (1962, 1979, 1991). Klagenfurt (2001: 140 ff., our translation) describes a central idea in the notion of polycontexturality as developed by Günther:

> By 'contexture' we understand a bivalently structured area that in a logical analysis could be considered to be a logical system of the classical bivalent logic. [...] A system is *polycontextural* if it consists of several contextures that are linked together through intermediating relations. [...] In the simplest case a polycontextural system consists of three contextures, which can, if necessary, increase its complexity by adding further contextures. As new contextures are added, other new contextures automatically emerge. These are called connection-contextures and mediate the new with the old contexture. Thus the individual contextures are ordered among themselves not hierarchically but heterarchically. Polycontexturality is therefore characterised by *intra*contexturality, the structural description of a contexture; *inter*contexturality, the description of the mediation between the individual contextures; and *discontexturality* as the description of the limits of contextures, among other aspects.

Polycontexturality means an excess of potential perspectives on a specific situation. But polycontexturality also implies that the different contextures are related to each other. Every contexture observes something but is also limited to a certain visual field. This limitation, blind spot or third element excluded in every distinction (the world, the unity of society, the observer) becomes the possible object of another observation observing in a different distinction. None of the chosen selections can claim finality over all others (Luhmann 1997a: 1132).

Seeing sociological potential in Günther's concept of polycontexturality, Luhmann transferred the logical meaning of polycontexturality into a sociological diagnosis and stated that, 'In our context polycontexturality shall mean that society develops numerous binary codes and programmes which depend on these' (1998: 666, our translation). Polycontexturality in the system-theoretical interpretation is not merely a set of epistemological assumptions according to which formally equal possibilities of different observations exist (Krause 1996: 143) but claims that society itself has become polycontextural with the emergence of functional differentiation. This sociological interpretation of polycontexturality involves the proposition that our society, especially in the transition from feudalism to modernity, has changed in such a way that polycontexturality itself is a prerequisite of modern communication.

A polycontextural society is a society with multiple binary codes and dependent programmes; it is a society that observes itself and its environment in different ways. Polycontexturality implies the simultaneous existence of different communicative codes, which, in turn, have different evaluative principles and different value systems. Polycontexturality is radical perspectivism in which the perspectives observe each other and relate to each other but also distance themselves to each other. Polycontexturality conceptualises not only the existence of different observations (binary codes) but also the mutual reflection of these various observations. The different contextures observe and depend on each other but without a common denominator on whose basis they can be compared – there are no hierarchical relations between the different observations. The arrangements of the contextures are heterarchical. This does not mean, however, that they are equal in the sense of equal importance or influence, but differences in degrees of domination need explanation since they do not simply exist as a natural condition.

If the diagnosis of a polycontextural society is correct, it will have consequences for maintaining social order. If a society is constituted by a multitude of different types of communication then sociologists must address the problem of why or how it is that incommensurable contextures do not lead to societies falling apart. A society with multiple observer positions needs techniques to relate these positions so that an arrangement arises that allows the different voices to coexist. It is this combination of discontexturality and intercontexturality that we refer to as multi-observer arrangements, understood as different types of constellations and configurations of contextures, observations and systems.[1] The essays in this book thus engage the cluster of ideas related to the concept of polycontexturality.

Polyphonic organisations

Where Luhmann talked about a polycontextural society, this book expands the idea and offers investigations of polycontexturality in relation to organisations. Systems theory distinguishes between function systems, organisations and interactions. These types of social systems refer to the different ways the communication structures itself. Function systems structure and define themselves by means of codes and programmes; interaction systems structure themselves by means of co-present and reflexively perceiving persons; and organisations structure themselves by means of members and decision premises (Luhmann 2000a). While Luhmann had a well-developed theory of societal differentiation, or of a polycontextural society (2012/13), he did not develop a concept of the polycontextural organisation. This was probably because he linked organisations and societal function systems too closely to one another (Kneer 2001).

Our point of departure is that health-care organisations today not only observe in a medical code but are able to actualise several codes in their observations and decision-making. For example, the work in a hospital is constantly potentially subject to financial, legal and medical observations and decisions. There are also issues relating to the education of the professional staff or to the occurrence of micro-political games. These matters all constitute different contextures, each of which depends on its own logic. This is also true for steering. According to Luhmann, to steer is to minimise a difference (for instance, between the budget and the expenditure); thus, different management programmes involve different types of observation (Luhmann 1997b). Contextures, however, are not just limited to formal management programmes; moral and political observations of an organisation, for example, can also form a contexture.

This raises questions regarding the relationships between the many potential contextures and organisational decision-making. For instance, what factors determine the contexture in which a decision is made? Is the decision about a given treatment observed as a medical, legal, financial, scientific or perhaps religious decision? Today, public and private organisations depend on money, but not all matters can be settled solely by reference to a financial code. We can analyse how the different contextures are actualised in decision-making, as well as how the relationships between different types of decisions and the contextures are regulated. We can analyse if there are any second-order contextures regulating when and how the different contextures are actualised. We can also discuss how some contextures become more important than others in the framing of the decision-making.

Andersen has suggested that the term 'polyphony', or 'heterophony', as he now prefers to call it, be introduced to conceptualise changes in the relationship between the links between organisations and function systems (Andersen 2003; Andersen and Born 2007; Thygesen and Andersen 2007). Polyphony refers to the phenomenon that organisational systems may be linked to several function systems with different types of communication. Polyphony can be seen as a special case of a polycontextural arrangement, namely as a situation where the distinction in which a decision is to be framed is undetermined: is it a medical decision, a financial decision, a legal decision or a political one? As Nassehi, Saake and Mayr point out in this book, it is nothing new that organisations work in reference to several function systems and their different codes. Thus, we suggest that the concept of polyphony be restricted to what can be termed 'unplanned' or 'indefinite' polycontextural decision-making. We can talk of polyphony if there are no fixed structures that determine in reference to which function system an organisational decision should be made or according to which function system it describes itself (such as an economic unit, a medical unit or some other unit).

The concept of polycontexturality renders it possible to make observations of indeterminacy as we are dealing not merely with separate logics or voices but with systems that observe each other and themselves – and that can make their actions dependent upon each other. Polycontexturality focuses attention on the different forms of observation taking place in the organisation, reflecting the fact that organisations observe in the context of several distinctions. This leads to issues regarding how organisations arrange their own polycontexturalities. In concrete empirical situations, we nevertheless encounter not just unspecified arrangements of voices but also specified ones. However they may work, these arrangements form orchestrated alignments of the different voices.

Some practices respond to this underlying problem of arranging incommensurable contextures. The differences between treatment practice and documentation, or between 'action and talk' as Brunsson (1989) puts it, may be utilised to cover up legally problematic treatment practices and provide an economically advantageous interpretation of the treatment. Corrupt and micro-political games can be compensated for by gossip. Likewise, transjunctional practices may prohibit the simultaneous presence of incommensurable contextures. Moreover, transcontextural semantics and practices may lead to the development of a complex of mutually conditioned contextures. For instance, thorough documentation of medical work could also be of administrative value and usable for accounting purposes, and thus it may regulate the relationship between the contextures.

Polycontexturality is potentially a problem concept, i.e. a concept that raises problems for which we may then seek solutions. Systems theory has several such problem concepts, such as complexity, double contingency and paradox. The role of these concepts is to inform the analyses in two ways. First, we have to specify in what sense we can talk about a problem, and, second, we have to identify what kinds of empirically developed solutions can solve the problem. In terms of a functional analysis (Luhmann 1970, 1995a: 52 ff.), we find that the concept of polycontexturality is associated with a methodology of formal analysis, 'which deals with the possibility of the possible' to see 'how the different possibilities bind each other, no matter what becomes real' (Esposito 2011: 133, our translation). As a problem concept of systems theory, polycontexturality points – as outlined above – to the dynamics, tensions and functions involved in multi-observer arrangements. With the concept of polycontexturality at its disposal, systems theory has gained conceptual tools that can be used to undertake a thorough examination of such functional arrangements – arrangements by which the different voices can come together in a working ecology. It is now possible to ask by means of what kind of practices the various contextures are linked and unlinked – and which arrangements emerge out of these practices. Polycontexturality yields to an order where reflections reflect on reflections and these reflections themselves promote the development of new reflective centres.

Current dynamics in relation to polycontexturality

Our diagnosis is that more and more codes of observation exist simultaneously. Different kinds of dynamics are involved in this current rearranging and intensification of polycontexturality. New kinds of regulation may create closer links between observations that have previously been only loosely connected. For instance, new kinds of financing may be introduced in an attempt to establish closer, more direct links between medical decisions and financial considerations. Reforms may be instituted with a view to forging closer ties between treatment, economising and patient satisfaction. Hospitals may import or invent new types of self-observation tailored to fit specific areas, such as production, finances, laws, patient satisfaction, prevention, quality. The reforms do not, we claim, negate or nullify the different contextures. They may, however, bring them closer to each other, not physically but in the sense that they become more relevant to each other (Vogd 2002; Knudsen 2007).

Another dynamic involved in the formation of multi-observer arrangements arises when social systems observe that they need other systems to achieve their own goals. For instance, health communication may observe that it needs educational communication to improve health. Another example would be in the event that the financial consequences of a medical decision are likely to have medical consequences in the future. In this case the medical system must also think in financial terms – for medical reasons. It may also be the other way round, for example, if the economy is given the responsibility of procuring as much health care as possible for the money available, then the economy must think about health care for financial reasons. Such situations demand an arrangement of different kinds of contextures. Polycontexturality can also mean that systems become *less* relevant to each other. Organisational systems such as hospitals and schools have traditionally had specific function systems (medicine and education) as the foundation of their decisions. If the organisation becomes more polycontextural, the links between organisations and specific function systems can become looser. This is then observed by the health professionals as managerialism and increasing financialisation of the hospital.

The different observations can exist simultaneously, but in organisations such as hospitals, different observations can be tested until a practical solution is found. When a patient in a unit for psychosomatic disorders threatens to disrupt procedures on the ward, then the treatment system may initially try conciliatory dialogue, and then resort to educative measures. If this does not help, then the patient may be pathologised, for example, based on the assumption that the root of the problem is a psychiatric issue. In the event of further resistance, legal semantics may come to the fore. In some cases, a relevant diagnosis may be stretched into the 'as if' mode to justify transferring the patient for psychiatric treatment.[2]

The systems may observe that they are dependent on each other but at the same time also observe that different observations carry different concerns and considerations. A decision that is medically correct can be problematic from a financial or legal point of view. A legally and financially correct decision may not be compatible with the rules of the medical profession. A medically correct proposal may be problematic because, if it were accepted, it might compromise the hierarchy between the senior doctors and the junior doctors. Similarly, no organisation can survive without respecting personal ambitions, even though this will sometimes be at the expense of profitability or foster illegal dealings, or even corrupt medical professionalism. Polycontexturality implicates a potentiality for conflicts and tensions.

Cognate theoretical perspectives

Various scholarly traditions work with issues and phenomena related to the ones that concern us here. In recent years, political science and sociology, in particular the sociology of organisations, have developed an increasing interest in the interplay between differences and incommensurabilites. This is reflected in concepts such as hybridisation (Hutter and Teubner 1993; Teubner 1996; Andersen and Sand 2012; Skelcher 2012), institutional logics (Lounsbury and Boxenbaum 2013), dissonance and heterarchy (Stark 2009) and the logics of justification (Boltanski and Thevenot 2006). The concepts of polyphony and institutional logics have both been highly prominent in discussions on various types of differentiations.

The concepts of polyphony and polyphonic organisations have developed particularly within narrative approaches to organisational analysis (Hazen 1993; Belova *et al.* 2008; Shotter 2008; Arnaboldi and Lapsley 2010; Belova 2010). Sullivan and McCarthy (2008: 525) define polyphony as follows: 'Broadly understood, polyphony has been used to refer to the multiple but equal voices that constitute organisations.' The interest in polyphony is related to what has been coined 'the linguistic turn'. Studies grounded in discourse theory have accorded a central position to polyphony (Carter *et al.* 2003; Kornberger *et al.* 2006). Kornberger *et al.* (2006: 8) offer the following definition: '[t]he polyphonic organisation is differentiated and constituted through different languages and rationalities'.

Another cognate branch of research is the neo-institutionalist research on institutional logics (see Thornton *et al.* 2012). In 1991, Friedland and Alford addressed the problem of multiple institutional references in detail. Their premise is 'that it is not possible to understand individual or organisational behaviour without locating it in a societal context' (1991: 232). Rather, they 'conceive of institutions as both supraorganisational patterns of activity through which humans conduct their material life in time and space, and symbolic systems, through which they categorize that activity and infuse it with meaning' (Friedland and Alford 1991: 232). The key point is that within an organisation various rationalities can exist simultaneously – for example, medical, political and economic – possibly expressing mutually contradictory logics. 'Each institutional order is both potentially autonomous and contradictory with others' (Friedland and Alford 1991: 259). But this does not imply that the individual institutional rationalities can exist independently of one another: 'The major institutions of contemporary society are interdependent and yet contradictory' (Friedland and Alford 1991: 256). Following the big tent approach (Lounsbury and Boxenbaum 2013: 5), a large number of papers on different notions of institutional logics are currently being produced (for instance, Volume 39A+B in *Research in the Sociology of Organisations*).

While we share an interest in non-hierarchical differentiations in organisational communication, we also see some conceptual problems in the two approaches mentioned. Narrative approaches to polyphony seem to risk conflating author, language, sentences, experience and intersubjectivity in the overly complex figure of the 'voice'. At the same time, the narrative approach to polyphony has difficulty with the unity of the polyphonic arrangement. Polyphony demands that we have a unit that is polyphonic. But what this unity is and how it relates to the different voices is not clear (Letiche 2010). Kornberger *et al.* pull the concept of polyphony in a more discursive direction. But this attempt also raises some questions with respect to the basic concepts. If the polyphonic organisation is differentiated on the basis of different languages (divided by 'gaps'), what then is *the* organisation? What is a 'language'? What kind of boundaries do we have between languages and what do they look like?

We share the intuition of institutional theory that modern society and its organisations are not characterised by identity but by difference. But the concept of institutional logics is, in our view, a very broad concept. It operates with *Kompaktbegriffe*, a German word that means compact concepts understood to hint at rather heterogeneous phenomena. The neo-institutional concept of institution is an example, where institution is often defined as practices, norms, values and assumptions.

The systems theory used in this book does not look for differences between institutional logics or between voices, but between observations. In the narrative tradition, polyphony is studied by following the 'authors' and their stories in the organisation. In a systems-theory perspective, in contrast, we look for observations; we do not follow the author, but the observer. In the narrative tradition, the identity of a voice is a person. In our communicative perspective, the human being is an addressee and an author in the communication – not a unity of voice, experience and body.[3] In our view, this conceptual choice sheds new light on well-known phenomena.

Our contention is that with systems theory and the concept of polycontexturality we can locate problematic issues and dynamics that are not observable within the frameworks of, for instance, institutional logics or narrative approaches to polyphony. The notions of institutional logics and polyphony illuminate and acknowledge the diversity of voices and logics. So does the notion of polycontexturality. But polycontexturality does something more. It points to the transjunctional (mediating) operations and practices that link observers together or that differentiate them from each other.

Chapters

The chapters in this book investigate different aspects of polycontexturality empirically. The book is divided into four parts related to different issues associated with polycontexturality. Below is a brief introduction to each topic and the related chapters.

Polycontextural constructions

It follows from the definition of polycontexturality that nothing is independent of observations. Polycontexturality refers to situations with multiple observations that inform and condition other observations in a recursive way. The first two chapters deal with this basic characteristic of polycontexturality as they analyse how drugs and bodies are subject to different observations and are hence constructed in diverse ways. Norms, values and political interests are areas in which we relatively easily accept that historical phenomena are socially constructed. But the two first chapters of this book demonstrate that such tangible phenomena as things (drugs) and bodies are also dependent on the observer. They also show how the different observations and their constructions may support each other – or may differentiate from each other.

Anna Henkel develops a polycontextural perspective on drugs. We already know from the placebo effect that drugs are not simply things that either exist or do not exist. Instead, they are polycontexturally constructed, as they depend on observation. Henkel shows how what is considered to be a drug changes with the emergence of a functionally differentiated society. In modernity, a drug was, for a while, relatively consistently regarded as something that served in medical treatment. But this arrangement is now being questioned. Instead, there are more and more things that insert themselves within a scientific and legal contexture and then claim to be extraordinarily effective and reliable but which do not claim to have a medical purpose. This is true of remedies that have little to do with medicine, such as herbicides and insecticides, but it is also true of such purposes that medicine has tried to keep outside of its purview for centuries, for example, agents for increasing strength, promoting reproduction and inducing abortions. Such products are no longer disqualified as quackery but are referred to as lifestyle products. Thus, polycontextural society creates functional arrangements that also allow multiple perspectives on the benefits and use of drugs. This creates uncertainty about what is to be considered medically necessary.

Holger Højlund and Anders la Cour investigate how residential institutions in Denmark have established various multi-observational arrangements for their inhabitants' physical bodies. Due to the inhabitants' psychological disadvantages, they cannot inform the residential care homes about their bodily needs. Instead, the residential care homes have to rely on an ever-increasing number of modern technologies that produce a range of different kinds of information about the condition of the body. The chapter demonstrates how these observations construct the body in various ways. These constructions create the necessary preconditions for the establishment of assorted social structures that link the body to the organisation. Finally, the chapter shows how the technologies make it possible for the otherwise silent bodily and psychological systems to become persons and thus connected to several function systems. These technologies thereby produce their own kind of polycontexturality of the body.

Societal arrangements

The chapters in Part II and in Part III deal with how different contextures are brought into a constellation with each other. The chapters by Werner Schirmer and Dimitris Michailakis and Niels Åkerstrøm Andersen and Hanne Knudsen deal with arrangements at a societal level. More specifically, they deal with prioritisation and responsibility under polycontextural conditions. With polycontexturality, the question is how a working arrangement of various contextures is created that avoids collision and ensures the continued autopoietic self-reproduction of the communicative systems.

The chapter by Andersen and Knudsen argues that hyper-responsibility emerges as a new form of personal responsibility equivalent to the emergence of heterophony. It focuses on the challenges the health system faces and how it ascribes responsibility to each individual. One of the current challenges for the health system is that it depends on non-health-related factors as it recognises that an individual's health depends not only on nutrition and exercise but also on socio-economic factors such as occupation, family and education. This makes it difficult for the health system to take responsibility for defining what personal responsibility for health includes. It in fact involves factors that are too numerous and too individual to be articulated as general rules or norms. In order to create a space for non-health-related perspectives, the health system calls for personal responsibility concerning health. The health system forces the individual to be a health subject while also simultaneously retracting this demand. It communicates the message that one should behave in healthy ways, but what 'healthy' means is up to oneself to decide, depending on one's life situation. A number of new technologies are being designed to communicate this 'both health and non-health' perspective. The chapter focuses on three specific technologies: health dialogues, health partnerships and health games, and the authors argue that these new technologies transmute personal responsibility into a hyper-responsibility equivalent to calling for heterophony.

The chapter by Schirmer and Michailakis describes how the welfare state tackles problems created by the need to set priorities in health care. It does this by reconciling the contradiction between the excluding nature of priority-setting and the integrity of its self-description as an inclusive welfare state. The goal is to find binding criteria for priority-setting that can be experienced as legitimate by everyone in spite of society's polycontextural structure. The authors argue that the polycontextural structure of modern society does not allow prioritisation on the societal level because there is no overarching or binding meta-criterion to justify decisions. The chapter analyses two different proposals that have been formulated to manage these health-policy issues. The proposals illustrate in two prototypical but opposing ways that prioritisation is impossible without some kind of hierarchy. The first proposal translates societal heterarchy into a primary hierarchy of principles for priority-setting in which political principles are superordinate to medical and economic ones. By contrast, the other proposal dissolves the hierarchy of principles and replaces it with a case-by-case evaluation left to a secondary hierarchy expressed by professional authority and formal organisation. The authors discuss how formal organisations can provide such a secondary hierarchy despite the heterarchical structure of a polycontextural society. With their recursive networks of decisions, formal organisations provide legitimate grounds for stratifying power and skills, thus creating space for case-by-case priority decisions. But this is not without tensions, as the polycontextural structure of modern society does not allow the development of a unitary or unifying set of criteria according to which prioritisations can be made. Ultimately, it does not matter which operational logic is followed, be it medical, economic, political or otherwise. In a polycontextural society, there will always be the legitimate possibility of applying yet another observational perspective from which the concrete priority-setting decision can be torpedoed.

Organisational arrangements

The papers in this section by Werner Vogd, Till Jansen and Sarah Poranzke and Daniel Lüdecke all deal with aspects of arrangements of different contextures in an organisation. They deal in particular with how arrangements are created between the areas of economics and medicine. Whereas institutional theory has focused mainly on how different 'logics' can coexist by coupling/uncoupling or by being loosely coupled (or by temporal sequentialisation), these chapters present different analyses of both problems and solutions related to polycontexturality.

Vogd's chapter deals with the arrangement of financial and medical demands in German hospitals. He focuses on concrete processes of treatment. Based on a detailed case analysis, Vogd shows that increasing financial pressure is not simply leading to reduced treatment quality. In particular, complex cases raise the issue of how the different logics of the function systems (particularly medicine, finance and law) can be brought together in a workable arrangement. An in-depth, longitudinal qualitative ethnographic study conducted on the medical ward of an urban German hospital demonstrates that it is no longer possible to achieve a balance between the requirements of medical practice and the financial demands by means of organisational management alone. Networks that cut across organisational boundaries are currently assuming an important function. They may also enable medical processes to be carried out when the treatment runs counter to the rational economic interests of the treating organisation.

Jansen and Poranzke focus on the position of clinical directors in German hospitals. Clinical directors are doctors by training but hold management positions where they have responsibility for both the medical treatment on their wards and for their financial results. Thus, the clinical directors are directly confronted with the challenge of bringing the medical and the financial contextures into an arrangement that works. Jansen and Poranzke's qualitative empirical study identifies three ways in which seemingly incommensurable perspectives can be brought into an arrangement. Their study clearly shows how many preconditions must be fulfilled to achieve a successful arrangement that comprises both the medical and financial aspects.

Lüdecke presents evidence for the importance and role of networks in the stabilisation of meaningful arrangements between different contextures. He begins by asking how sustainable work alliances can be formed in integrated care. Taking into account the basic conflict between the medical and financial systems, he examines the question as to what control mechanisms are applied to make arrangements within these polycontextural conditions. To investigate this issue, Lüdecke employed qualitative interviews with actors involved in interface management and integrated-care partnerships (e.g., hospital discharge). He demonstrates that loosely linked networks can take on important control functions in the sustainable balancing of financial, nursing and medical demands. On the other hand, it becomes clear that if

the links are too tightly forged, the extreme case being an insurance company with a quasi-monopoly, it hampers the dynamic balancing and relating
of different contextures. In this case the actors working at the interface lose
the autonomy necessary to be able to find the best solutions in the specific
situation.

Reflections

Social systems are systems that observe themselves and other social systems. The chapters in this section deal with how polycontextural social systems observe their own polycontexturality – and what implications this has.
Related to the issue of self-observation is the issue of self-description. One
example is the development of new types of semantics for reflection, for
example, ethical communication. We also see parasitic codification when
politicians, for instance, use references to scientific evidence in a political
communication (Stäheli 1996).

The chapter by Armin Nassehi, Irmhild Saake and Katharina Mayr deals
with ethical discourses, which is an interesting area of investigation when
it comes to polycontextural arrangements. On the one hand, ethical discourses have their origin in relatively specialised scientific and philosophical
reflections, while, on the other, they are also considered to be independent
voices in political and health-related organisations. According to Nassehi
et al.'s findings, health-care ethics committees (HECs) are faced with the
structural impossibility of generating a total perspective from various professional and practical perspectives. When it comes to the differing logics of
science, nursing, medicine, law and economics, decisions cannot be made
on the basis of a principle of consensus. Ethics committees cannot establish
consensus. The findings of their study, however, show that they do something else: they ensure that different voices are heard – and that if one voice
is heard, this does not necessarily mean that another voice will be negated.
The incommensurability of different forms of practice and different perspectives for reflection is not only recognised but also welcomed in HECs. Thus,
the claim of this chapter is that the functional significance of HECs is that
they help an organisation to deal with the multiplicity of speaker positions
by establishing islands inside the organisations where these may be visible
not as absolute truths but precisely *as* speaker positions.

Barry Gibson and Jennifer Burr are also concerned with ethics. Their
chapter takes as its starting point the development of increasingly special-
ist communication about ethics in scientific research. Drawing on the work
of Luhmann, it proposes that we can study communication about research
ethics as an empirical phenomenon. In doing so, it follows Luhmann's work
stipulation to treat the norms of ethics within scientific research as facts. In
doing so, the authors explore when norms are successful at conditioning
communication and where they are suspended. The chapter is based on the
study of organisational communications about research ethics and uncovers

how ethical communication seeks to preserve the subject status of research participants as subjects. The authors also discuss how several other distinctions, including the human and non-human distinction and the benefit and harm distinction, are deployed and suspended in ethical communication. The chapter also explores how these distinctions encounter each other and are handled in very different ways according to the contexture in which they are used. The comparison of communication between different organisational contextures, such as how each organisational contexture sees the environment of its research, has enormous consequences for the application of ethical distinctions in such communication.

The chapter by Morten Knudsen interprets the currently increasing emphasis on leadership and the emergence of leadership semantics in hospital settings as a reflection of changing social structures leading to new conditions for the inclusion of managers in organisations. The argument is that the current semantics of personal leadership in health-care organisations (and other public organisations) reflect the polyphony of the organisations. In the polyphonic organisation the manager finds many roles but no organisationally given unified position. This is reflected in the semantics that articulate the person as something external to the organisation that endows the manager with his or her unique power. The study's findings reveal that this exclusion of the manager from the organisation is compensated for by means of management training, leadership development and the like.

Combined, the chapters provide a broad-based analysis of the dynamics and complexities of polycontextural conditions. They throw new light on how the differentiations between communicative codes and programmes and how the formation of new types of arrangements between them are interwoven. The authors demonstrate how the contextures can observe each other and reflect on their own boundaries. They may take part in common constructions (of drugs, for instance), while at the same time the constructions are observed in different ways: for example, drugs are continually being observed differently by different systems. The contextures have an interest in each other; however, this does not lead to compromises or to the disappearance of differences. The differences are not reconciled, but they can become part of complex arrangements. The obligation of health-care systems to treat diseases does not disappear because new financial instruments and market mechanisms are introduced. No new rationality uniting the medical and financial rationalities is revealed. Instead, we can investigate how society and its organisations must simultaneously manage contextures that do not fit together. The differences between them are maintained at the same time as they are all arranged with and connected to each other. Instead of having to arrive at compromises or reconciliations of differences, the systems-theory approach makes it possible to insist on boundaries and closed systems, which can nonetheless observe each other and form different types of complex arrangements.

Notes

1 See Vogd 2010 for a more in-depth discussion of the concept of societal polycontexturality.
2 For a detailed case analysis, see Vogd (2004: 365 ff.).
3 On a psychological level, this parallels the social psychological finding of a post-modern self, understood more as a multiple entity than as a unit (cf. Gergen 1991).

References

Andersen, N. Å. (2003) 'Polyphonic Organisations', in T. Hernes and T. Bakken (eds.) (2003) *Autopoietic Organization Theory*, Oslo: Abstrakt, Liber, Copenhagen Business School Press, pp. 151–82.
Andersen, N. Å. and A. Born (2007) 'Heterophony and the Postponed Organisation: Organizing Autopoietic Organisations', *Tamara Journal*, 6 (2): 176–86.
Andersen, N. Å. and I. J. Sand (eds.) (2012) *Hybrid Forms of Governance: Self-suspension of Power*, Basingstoke: Palgrave Macmillan.
Arnaboldi, M. and I. Lapsley (2010) 'Asset Management in Cities: Polyphony in Action?', *Accounting Auditing and Accountability Journal*, 23 (3): 392–419.
Baraldi, C., G. Corsi and E. Esposito (1997) *GLU: Glossar zu Niklas Luhmanns Theorie sozialer Systeme*, Frankfurt: Suhrkamp.
Belova, O. (2010) 'Polyphony and the Sense of Self in Flexible Organizations', *Scandinavian Journal of Management*, 26 (1): 67–76.
Belova, O., I. King and M. Sliwa (2008) 'Introduction: Polyphony and Organization Studies: Mikhail Bakhtin and Beyond', *Organization Studies*, 29 (4): 493–500.
Boltanski, L. and L. Thévenot (2006) *On Justification: Economies of Worth*, Princeton, NJ: Princeton University Press.
Borch, C. (2011) *Niklas Luhmann*, London and New York: Routledge.
Bourdieu, P. (1998) *Practical Reason: On the Theory of Action*, Palo Alto, Calif.: Stanford University Press.
Brunsson, N. (1989) *Organisation of Hypocrisy: Talk, Decisions and Actions in Organisations*, Chichester: Wiley.
Carter, C., S. Clegg, J. Hogan and M. Kornberger (2003) 'The Polyphonic Spree: The Case of the Liverpool Dockers', *Industrial Relations*, 34 (4): 290–304.
Durkheim, É. (1984) *The Division of Labour in Society*, New York: The Free Press.
Esposito, E. (2011) 'Kann Kontingenz formalisiert werden?', *Soziale Systeme*, 17 (1): 120–37.
Foucault, M. (2003) *The Birth of the Clinic: An Archaeology of Medical Perception*, London and New York: Routledge.
Friedland, R. and R. Alford (1991) 'Bringing Society Back In: Symbols, Practices, and Institutional Contradictions', in W. W. Powell and P. J. DiMaggio (eds.), *The New Institutionalism in Organisational Analysis*, Chicago, Ill.: University of Chicago Press, pp. 232–66.
Gergen, K. (1991) *The Saturated Self: Dilemmas of Identity in Contemporary Life*, New York: Basic Books.
Günther, G. (1962) 'Cybernetic Ontology and Transjunctional Operations', in M. C. Yovits, G. T. Jacobi and G. D. Goldstein (eds.), *Self-organizing Systems*, Washington, DC: Spartan Books, pp. 313–92.

——(1979) 'Life as Polycontexturality', in G. Günther (ed.), *Beiträge zur Grundlegung einer operationsfähigen Dialektik*, vol. II, Hamburg: Meiner, pp. 283–306.

——(1991) *Idee und Grundriß einer nicht-Aristotelischen Logik: Die Idee und ihre philosophischen Voraussetzungen*, Hamburg: Meiner.

Habermas, Jürgen (1988) *Theorie des kommunikativen Handelns: Zweiter Band*, Frankfurt: Suhrkamp.

Harste, G. (2013) 'The Big, Large and Huge Case of State-Building: Studying Structural Coupling at the Macro Level', in A. Febbrajo and G. Harste (eds.), *Law and Intersystemic Communication: Understanding 'Structural Coupling'*, London: Ashgate, pp. 67–96.

Hazen, M. A. (1993) 'Towards Polyphonic Organizations', *Journal of Organizational Change Management*, 6 (5): 15–26.

Hutter, M. and G. Teubner (1993) 'The Parasitic Role of Hybrids', *Journal of Institutional and Theoretical Economics/Zeitschrift für die gesamte Staatswissenschaft*, 149 (4): 706–15.

Jahraus, O., A. Nassehi, M. Grizelj, I. Saake, C. Kirchmeier and J. Müller (2012) *Luhmann Handbuch: Leben-Werk-Wirkung*, Stuttgart: J. B. Metzler.

Klagenfurt, K. (2001) *Technologische Zivilisation und transklassische Logik. Eine Einführung in die Technikphilosophie Gotthard Günthers*, Frankfurt: Suhrkamp.

Kneer, G. (2001) 'Organisation und Gesellschaft: Zum ungeklärten Verhältnis von Organisations und Funktionssystemen in Luhmanns Theorie sozialer Systeme', *Zeitschrift für Soziologie*, 30 (6): 407–28.

Knudsen, M. (2007) 'Structural Couplings Between Organizations and Function Systems: Looking at Standards in Health Care', *Cybernetics and Human Knowing*, 14 (2–3): 111–31.

——(2010) 'Surprised by Method: Functional Method and Systems Theory', *Forum Qualitative Sozialforschung/Forum: Qualitative Social Research*, 11 (3).

Kornberger, M., S. Clegg and C. Carter (2006) 'Rethinking the Polyphonic Organisation: Managing as Discursive Practice', *Scandinavian Journal of Management*, 22 (1): 3–30.

Krause, D. (1996) *Luhmann-Lexikon: eine Einführung in das Gesamtwerk von Niklas Luhmann mit 25 Abbildungen und über 400 Stichworten*, Stuttgart: Ferdinand Enke Verlag.

Letiche, Hugo (2010): 'Polyphony and Its Other', *Organization Studies*, 31 (3): 261–77.

Lounsbury, M. and E. Boxenbaum (2013) 'Institutional Logics in Action', *Research in the Sociology of Organisations*, 39A: 3–22.

Luhmann, N. (1970) 'Funktionale Methode und Systemtheorie', in *Soziologische Aufklärung 2*, Opladen: Westdeutscher Verlag.

——(1979) *Trust and Power*, Chichester: Wiley.

——(1980) *Gesellschaftsstruktur und Semantik: Studien zur Wissenssoziologie der modernen Gesellschaft. Band 1*, Frankfurt: Suhrkamp.

——(1983a) 'Anspruchsinflation im Krankheitssystem. Eine Stellungnahme aus gesellschaftstheoretische Sicht', in P. Herder-Dorneich and A. Schuller (eds.), *Die Anspruchsspirale: Schicksal oder Systemdefekt?* Stuttgart: Kohlhammer, pp. 28–49.

——(1983b). 'Medizin und Gesellschaftstheorie', *Medizin Mensch Gesellschaft*, 8: 168–75.

——(1987) *Soziologische Aufklärung 4: Beiträge zur funktionalen Differenzierung der Gesellschaft*, Opladen: Westdeutscher Verlag.

——(1988) *Soziale Systeme. Grundriss einer allgemeinen Theorie*, Frankfurt: Suhrkamp.

——(1989) *Ecological Communication*, Chicago, Ill.: University of Chicago Press.

——(1990a) *Die Wirtschaft der Gesellschaft*, Frankfurt: Suhrkamp.

——(1990b) 'Der medizinische Code', in *Soziologische Aufklärung 5*, Opladen: Westdeutscher Verlag, pp. 176–88.

——(1993) *Risk: A Sociological Theory*, Berlin: de Gruyter.

——(1995a) *Social Systems*, Stanford, Calif.: Stanford University Press.

——(1995b) *Das Recht der Gesellschaft*, Frankfurt: Suhrkamp. Published in English in 2004 as *Law as a Social System*, Oxford: Oxford University Press.

——(1995c) *Die Kunst der Gesellschaft*, Frankfurt: Suhrkamp. Published in English in 2000 as *Art as a Social System*, Palo Alto, Calif.: Stanford University Press.

——(1996a) *Die Wirtschaft der Gesellschaft*, Frankfurt: Suhrkamp.

——(1996b) *Die Realität der Massenmedien, 2., erweiterte Auflage*, Opladen: Westdeutscher Verlag. Published in 2000 as *The Reality of the Mass Media*, Cambridge: Polity Press.

——(1997a): *Die Gesellschaft der Gesellschaft*, Frankfurt: Suhrkamp. Published in 2012/13 as *Theory of Society*, 2 vols., Palo Alto, Calif.: Stanford University Press.

——(1997b) 'Limits of Steering', *Theory, Culture and Society*, 14 (1): 41–57.

——(1998) *Die Wissenschaft der Gesellschaft*, Frankfurt: Suhrkamp.

——(2000a) *Organisation und Entscheidung*, Opladen: Westdeutscher Verlag.

——(2000b) *Die Politik der Gesellschaft*, Frankfurt: Suhrkamp.

——(2000c) *Die Religion der Gesellschaft*, Frankfurt: Suhrkamp

——(2002) *Das Erziehungssystem der Gesellschaft*, Frankfurt: Suhrkamp.

——(2012–13) *Theory of Society*, 2 vols., Stanford, Calif.: Stanford University Press.

Marx, K. (1989) *Das Kapital: Kritik der politischen Ökonomie*, Berlin: Dietz Verlag.

Moeller, H. G. (2006) *Luhmann Explained: From Souls to Systems*, Chicago, Ill.: Open Court.

——(2012) *The Radical Luhmann*, New York: Columbia University Press.

Parsons, T. (1979) *The Social System*, London: Routledge & Kegan Paul Ltd.

Schimank, U. (2007) *Theorien gesellschaftlicher Differenzierung*, Wiesbaden: VS Verlag für Sozialwissenschaften.

Shotter, J. (2008) 'Dialogism and Polyphony in Organizing Theorizing in Organization Studies: Action Guiding Anticipations and the Continuous Creation of Novelty', *Organization Studies*, 29 (4): 501–24.

Simmel, G. (1989) *Über sociale Differenzierung, Gesamtausgabe Band 2*, Frankfurt: Suhrkamp.

Skelcher, C. (2012) 'What Do We Mean When We Talk About 'Hybrids' and 'Hybridity' in Public Management and Governance?' Working Paper, Institute of Local Government Studies, Birmingham: University of Birmingham.

Spencer Brown, G. (1972) *Laws of Form*, New York: Julian.

Stäheli, U. (1996) 'From Victimology Towards Parasitology: The Function of Exclusion', *Recherches Sociologiques*, 27 (2): 59–80.

Stark, D. (2009) *The Sense of Dissonance: Accounts of Worth in Economic Life*, Princeton, NJ: Princeton University Press.

Stollberg, G. 2009 'Das medizinische System: Überlegungen zu einem von der Soziologie vernachlässigten Funktionssystem', *Soziale Systeme*, 15 (1): 189–217.

Sullivan, P. and J. McCarthy (2008) 'Managing the Polyphonic Sounds of Organizational Truths', *Organization Studies*, 29 (4): 525–42.

Teubner, G. (1996) 'Double Bind: Hybrid Arrangements as De-paradoxifiers', *Journal of Institutional and Theoretical Economics/Zeitschrift für die gesamte Staatswissenschaft*, 151 (1): 59–64.

Thornton, P. H., W. Ocasio and M. Lounsbury (2012) *The Institutional Logics Perspective: A New Approach to Culture, Structure and Process*, Oxford: Oxford University Press.

Thygesen, N. T. and N. Å. Andersen (2007) 'The Polyphonic Effects of Technological Changes in Public Sector Organizations: A System Theoretical Approach', *Ephemera*, 7 (2): 326–45.

Vogd, W. (2002) 'Professionalisierungsschub oder Auflösung ärztlicher Autonomie?' *Zeitschrift für Soziologie*, 31 (4): 294–315.

——(2004) *Ärztliche Entscheidungsprozesse des Krankenhauses im Spannungsfeld von System- und Zweckrationalität*, Berlin: Verlag für Wissenschaft und Forschung.

——(2005) 'Medizinsystem und Gesundheitswissenschaften: Rekonstruktion einer schwierigen Beziehung', *Soziale Systeme*, 11 (2): 236–70.

——(2010) *Systemtheorie und rekonstruktive Sozialforschung: Eine empirische Versöhnung unterschiedlicher theoretischer Perspektiven*, Opladen: Barbara Budrich.

White, K. (2009) *An Introduction to the Sociology of Health and Illness*, London: Sage.

Part I

Polycontextural constructions

1 Drugs in modern society

Analysing polycontextural things under the condition of functional differentiation

Anna Henkel

The endeavour of this chapter is to offer a way for analysing drugs in modern society. The importance of drugs is, on the one hand, obvious: they produce measurable effects, they create costs for the health-insurance companies, and they probably share significantly in the esteem the medical profession has enjoyed for the past two thousand years. On the other hand, there is a problem: in view of the historical development of what is deemed a drug as well as the evolution of corresponding medical and natural scientific theories, 'drugs' can hardly be considered a consistent category. So what are drugs? This issue is further complicated by the fact that sociology does not usually pay much attention to the analysis of seemingly non-social objects such as 'drugs' or the relationship between society and the construction of things.

Despite the neglect of issues in sociological thinking, I will show that drugs are not simply neutral objects with given qualities but do stand in a certain relationship to medical action and communication. Furthermore, I will show how this relationship changes between the social constitution of drugs and communication with regard to medical treatment as society is transformed. Reviewing the history of pharmaceuticals, it becomes obvious that almost everything was seen as a drug at one time: from cabbage in the old Roman Empire and the fat of people hanged in the Middle Ages to certain fungi in modern society (penicillin). Given this variety, it seems worthwhile to correlate society and the distinct issues it dealt with, and, at the same time, we might learn something about this society if we take its things into consideration.

In the first two sections, this chapter provides a concept of society and a concept of drugs as starting points for the analysis that follows. These starting points are detailed in the following three sections, on the relationship between society and drugs, on current discussions on placebos and functional foods, and the relationship between drugs and organisation. The last section offers some perspectives on the importance of analysing things for the theory of society.

Conceptualise society: functional differentiation and polycontexturality

A main idea of this chapter is that what constitutes drugs changes with the evolution of society. Because we aim to obtain a clearer understanding of drugs in modern society, it is important to first get a notion of modern society. This section briefly describes the concept of modern society as a functionally differentiated society. Polycontexturality is shown to be a specific consequence from functional differentiation.

A main characteristic of modern society is its particular type of differentiation. Despite the existence of other striking characteristics, such as Weber's idea of rationalisation or the modern idea of a knowledge society, different sociological approaches can at least agree to describe modern society as a differentiated society. This description is important in Weber's value-spheres (1920/1988: 244 ff.) as well as in Mead's consideration of a functional differentiation of human society through language (1967: 244, 288 ff., 326 ff.) or in perspectives of action theory (Schimank 2007) and is equally reflected in systems-theory concepts (Luhmann 1999).

Luhmann observes modern society primarily as a functionally differentiated society. His notion of functional differentiation implies that communication is no longer primarily oriented as a social hierarchy but follows self-referential selection criteria of meaning contexts (i.e. codes of functional systems). Law is not what a God defines as law but what, according to the criteria of the legal system, can be seen as lawful instead of unlawful. The same is true for science, economics, religion and several further value-spheres. Luhmann examined such specificities of functional differentiation. I will therefore simply provide a synthesis: in a theory that defines the social as self-referential communication, modern society is mainly characterised by its functional systems in the sense of self-referential contexts of meaning.

There are, of course, a lot of consequences from this perspective on society. For the purposes of this chapter I would like to draw attention only to one of them: the *polycontexturality* of perspectives that evolves with functional differentiation. Under the condition of functional differentiation, each functional system develops its own specific construction of a topic. As a result, there is not only one perspective on a certain topic but a number of different but equally valuable perspectives.

Take unforeseen side effects of drugs as an example. From the perspective of *science*, the possibility of side effects is not a risk but a fact constitutive for how science is operating; it is the idea of science to produce new facts, until now anything is seen as potentially harbouring an undisclosed issue. This at first neutral situation becomes a risk from the *medical* point of view: a medical treatment might shift from making someone healthy to making them sick – and this is a risk because it (as scientific progress) is outside the medical system. For the *political* system, the scientific fact of possible side effects, and the medical risk of causing illness, can mean the risk of political scandal. The side effects of drugs were not a part of the political discourse for a very long time. Even the Thalidomide scandal in the 1950s, a drug that caused severe birth defects, had almost no political repercussions at all. Only a second scandal involving a dietary product shortly afterwards transformed side effects into a political issue. Finally, from an *economic* point of view, the risk of side effects means a drop in profits. The same issue, possible unforeseen side effects of drugs, thus produces very different risks depending on the context.

In a functionally differentiated society, the terminology of polycontexturality in the aftermath of Gotthardt Günther can be applied regarding this specific relation of observation. The concept of polycontexturality in the first step refers to the level of society. It points to the fact that topics and situations can be reconstructed from different contexts of viewpoints, with consequences such as a competition of interpretational offers or mutual self-irritation or such interpretive self-irritation of these different communicational logics (Vogd 2010). The idea of polycontexturality is at the same time a logical and empirical hypothesis on society. The *logical* hypothesis states that a two-valued logic must be replaced by a three-valued logic so as to adequately account for the phenomenon of self-reference and its implied dimension of time. The *empirical* hypothesis states that society creates polycontextural relations of observation when it moves into a state of functional differentiation. Despite the fact that communication generally is thought of as recursive, polycontexturality remains the specific perspective of observation of a functionally differentiated society.

Conceptualise drugs: the drug as structural identity

In the first section we gained a starting point for the analysis of drugs in modern society by discussing the notion of modern society: modern society can be observed as functionally differentiated, with the consequence of polycontexturality regarding important issues of society. Before we can start our core analysis of drugs in modern society, we now, as a second starting point, have to develop a concept of drugs consistent with our notion of modern society. Obviously, an ontological understanding of drugs is not compatible with the notion of polycontexturality. I will argue that it is useful to conceptualise drugs as structural identities that are characterised by the (potentially changing) expectations attached to them.

A new sociology of medical treatment would not be complete if it did not take drugs into account. Since Hippocrates, medical treatment with the means of drugs is one of the three medical pillars, next to dietary and surgical means (Schmitz 1998; Schulze 2002). No small part of the reputation of the first medical practitioners is due not to the surgical and artisanal aptitude of their knowledge about a balanced way of living (the word 'diet' comes from the Greek word for *way of living*), but their reputation is due to the rational medical application of pharmaceuticals (in Greek the word for medical potions) which before then only priests could provide. Drug treatment has become the predominant means of healing, which proved functionally equivalent to other ways of medical treatment, including surgical measures (Friedrich *et al.* 1977; Rosenbrock and Gerlinger 2006).

Obviously, drugs are an important issue for the sociology of medical treatment. That further begs the question of whether drugs should be treated analytically with regards to a polycontextural perspective. Within social research in general, drugs are an issue that is rarely addressed (for an overview, see Abraham 2008; Henkel 2012). Taking polycontexturality as the research perspective, current approaches to observing drugs become difficult to apply, like a focus on the interests and power especially of the pharmaceutical industry on drug development (Abraham 2010) or a focus on the prescription attitudes of doctors (Lilja 1976). What remains is to use drugs themselves as the relevant reference point, as the tertium comparationis (Vogd 2010: 31) of polycontextural observation and to ask how this approach may contribute to a new sociology of medical treatment.

To make the 'drug' itself the *tertium comparationis* of polycontextural constructions incurs – at least at first – conceptual difficulties. At the core of these difficulties, especially from a perspective of system theory, is the consideration that drugs are *things* and accordingly cannot be observed as self-referential systems like society or organisation. On the contrary: things appear to be entirely beyond the object of research as defined by systems theory within sociology.[1] This consideration might be the reason why there was no analytical perspective on 'things' that developed in the context of systems theory and that empirical studies on 'things' are equally a desideratum.[2] The theoretical reservations with regard to things betrays itself in remarks according to which the research of self-referential systems required a logic of three values, while the research of things might content itself with a logic of two values (Vogd 2010: 46): a thing is, or it is not. The example of the placebos indicates that this distinction is too easy. In this case, the thing is and is not a drug at the same time, depending on the observer.

A dichotomy of self-referential systems of meaning on the one side and two-value based objective things on the other is not compatible with the general starting point of the social as communication. Meaning in this theory is conceptualised as the last horizon (*Letzthorizont*); non-meaning is not accessible. We therefore cannot make any 'true' declaration about a possible observer-independent objectiveness of a being or thing as such. What is accessible for sociological research is only that which under certain social conditions successfully claims to be the true reconstruction of the world 'outside' of social meaning. From this perspective, approaches which claim a quasi-social influence of the non-meaningful by its *materiality* are to be doubted (see, e.g., Hacking 1983; Pickering 1989; Latour 1995). Instead, we are interested in *how society constructs the non-meaningful* and *how the forms of the meaningful and description of the non-meaningful change as society changes*. From the perspective of system theory's notion of society, we can apply as a heuristic hypothesis that the social construction of the non-meaningful and probably even the function of such constructions changes with the evolution to a functionally differentiated, polycontextural society.

Things themselves are not reflexive. But *how* they *really* are is not accessible to communication. Accessible is only their communicative reconstruction. In other places I demonstrated that drugs can be analysed sociologically by means of the analytical category of the pharmacon with regard to the semantical and social evolution of the pharmaceutical (Henkel 2011, 2012, 2013). With regard to the new sociology of medical treatment endeavoured in this publication, I apply the research perspective of polycontexturality to the empirical case of the drug.

Accordingly, there are three analytical questions from the general approach which I review here: first, what it means for drugs to be considered as a *tertium comparationis*; second, which contextures of this *tertium comparationis* relate to each other; and third, which relation persists regarding a polycontextural organisation. *The tertium comparationis of this contribution is the drug in the sense that 'drug' as a reference point remains identical, but is embedded in different discursive contexts.* How can such a reference point be further understood?

A non-meaningful environment is real for communication in so far as it has been through the double filter of consciousness and communication. This meaningful construction of the non-meaningful is based on attributions of expectations. What remains is the by-no-means-unimportant question of *what* such expectations are attributed to. Luhmann, in this context, considers things as structural identities, analogous to persons, roles, programmes and values which equally attract expectations and make them durable by themselves persisting as an identity (1984: 424 ff.). In the case of roles, programmes and values, it may remain plausible to understand such identities as communicative structures. But already, when persons are concerned, the body is forced upon the observer as something going beyond communication. This is all the more true in the case of the thing and its material substance. Yet, concerning persons, Luhmann himself explained that in this case the communicative structure provides the reference identity (2005b). In an analogous way, it is true for things: a body or material substrate does not procure the structural identity but rather a communicative structure.

Analogous to the role of the doctor or the value of human dignity, a *drug therefore is considered a structural identity, which is characterised by the expectations in it*. A specific aspect of these expectations is that they are attached to a non-meaningful entity and give themselves a non-reflexive form, while at the same time these constructions stem from a reflexive social process and accordingly must be considered as reflexive expectations. The social construction of drugs also is the construction of social expectations regarding drugs, which implies the expectation that we are concerned with a non-meaningful entity. The drug does not communicate itself what one is supposed to do, and it is not important to understand the drug for its being effective – so far at least as the scientific description, which observes drugs as an objective reality. But even such a (two-valued) position of observation must be and is disrupted by the phenomenon of the placebo, a case in which the thing itself remains, from a scientific point of view, without effectiveness. In a social theory that accepts differentiation and polycontexturality, this phenomenon of the placebo can be explained by the set of expectations that stem from different social contextures.

From cosmos to contextures: changing constructions of drugs

In the first two sections we gained a notion of modern society as functionally differentiated and a concept of drugs as *tertium comparationis*, which does not define properties of drugs but refers to them as structural identities which are characterised by the expectations in them. Now, let us put these two points together and start the main part of the analysis of drugs in modern society. In this section I will show how the notion of a drug has changed over the course of history and the evolution of society. In antique and medieval society, drugs were observed as ontological entities with a distinct place in a medical-philosophical idea of a cosmos. In modern, differentiated society, attributing something as a drug requires the coherent interaction between the construction of different contextures. Natural sciences, technology, law/politics, medicine and pharmaceuticals create drug constructions on their own terms; only when all of these factors work together can one undisputedly call something a drug.

Central for drugs as non-meaningful things is the context in which the expectation of materiality attributed to the drug develops. Though the term 'materiality' immediately evokes an idea of constancy and inalterability, there is a fundamental change in the reasons given for such a constant and in the notion of what materiality is. For centuries, the idea of materiality was rooted in the antique philosophy of a *balanced cosmos*. With regard to drugs, it was up to medicine to apply the general notion of balance. The gist of this medical-philosophical idea of drugs is that the four elements (water, fire, earth and sky) are related to the four bodily fluids. The body is healthy when these four fluids are in equilibrium. Pharmaca are used when the body is out of balance. Since everything in the cosmos implies four elements, a warming pharmacon may, for example, rebalance a cold body.

For a long time, the materiality of drugs was thought of in terms of equilibration and cosmic elements and was thus regarded from the world view in which medicine is seen as a part of a general cosmology. With the development of *modern natural sciences*, this conception of materiality dissolves and, with it, the theoretical context of how drugs should be perceived. Medicine reinvented itself in terms of the new scientific notion of the body. But when it comes to the concept of drugs, the medical contexture loses its defining power. With the differentiation of medicine and natural science, it is now the scientific contexture instead of the medical one that constructs the relevant categories for the observation of drugs. The notion of substance is replaced by the notion of chemical active substances. No longer is the whole plant or mineral considered to be medically effective because of its balancing effect to an unbalanced body. Instead, the effectiveness of drugs is considered to be down to certain chemical elements and their scientific properties.

This shift to a natural understanding of materiality based upon the natural sciences has consequences for the *technological contextualisation* of drugs. As long as the entire plant is supposed to be effective due to its elementary mixture, the entire plant must be used for medical treatment. Accordingly, the predominant way a drug was administered was the potion: the fresh ingredients were dried and later boiled in water or dissolved in wine. The techniques were strenuous but did not require a lot of knowledge. This changed with the shift to active substances. A separate technological contexture becomes relevant to extract or gain active substances. Already in the early development of active-substance pharmacy, pharmaceutical techniques became a separate field of knowledge. While the main task in earlier times was to correctly recognise and store the ingredients of drugs, now difficult (al-)chemical procedures become necessary for gaining active substances. With the success of the active-substance paradigm, technical requirements become so high that the pharmacy as the traditional place for manufacturing drugs could no longer keep up with the complexity of developments. Technology is not only important for gaining active substances but also for the development of applicable drug forms. Because active substances are highly effective even in very small doses – other than the traditional potions – new drug forms are required which are exact and easy to administer. The technology of compression, derived from the manufacturing of charcoal, is applied to drugs, and the tablet as a new delivery vehicle was invented at the end of the nineteenth century. The tablet was extremely important for the shift from traditional potions to new active-substance drugs.

With the innovation of the tablet, drugs lasted longer, were easier to transport and could be given in exact doses. At the same time, the individual preparation was replaced by a *standardised product*. Apart from the natural scientific description and the use of active substances, technological possibilities of producing the final product became important. The successful development of drugs as active-substance-based ready-made drugs requires the combination of technical and scientific knowledge: a tiny mistake can make active substances lethal – the drug is dependent on a technically enabled, simple dose.

Furthermore, the meaningful construction of the non-meaningful identity of the modern drug implies a *legal context*. Just as in the scientific and technical context, the legal context lays out what is considered as a drug. Drug laws accordingly define the range of application. In this way, the law regulated which requirements had to be fulfilled for something to be considered a drug. At the same time, the legal context 'individualises' drugs. Patent and trademark protection laws create the legal construction for drugs as packaged ready-made drugs. To be legally sold to a consumer, active substances of a drug must fulfill certain legal requirements, and the drug itself must be packaged with information on its name, ingredients, the name and address of the producer, how many pills, etc.

Between the natural scientific, technical and legal contexts, there is a *recursive relationship of mutual services*: to define its area of application, the legal context falls back on natural scientific criteria and technically enabled forms of individualisation. Because legally required tests become a condition for putting a drug on the market, the legal and scientific sides again work together. The research on regulation of knowledge in similar cases speaks of 'reflexive regulation' (Schuppert and Voßkuhle 2008; Bora 2009). The law takes up scientific definitions for its own definitions and influences the development of scientific knowledge by requiring non-scientific purposes such as health or the lack of risk.

The drug as a semantic identity works as a structural coupling of different contextures, which each in their specific context of meaning define the identity of the drug. Due to the common relation to the identical term drug, these constructions of different contextures may irritate each other. This identity enacts functional systems and procures their co-evolution in a polycontextural society.

Another important contexture for the construction of drugs is *medicine*. Though no longer important regarding the definition of the material gist of drugs, the medical contexture is relevant for the construction of the expectations regarding the specific effectiveness of drugs. With the natural scientific definition of an active substance's identity, no reasons for any medical effectiveness are given. On the contrary: natural scientific findings are characterised by the fact that they can potentially create effectiveness to *different* ends. To create the medical effectiveness of drugs, three contextures are involved: the natural-scientific, the legal, and the medical.

Compared to medieval medicine, which was rooted in philosophy, the basis of medicine profoundly changed. The notion of the body and its health is now related to natural scientific ideas instead of an idea of a balanced cosmos. In the context of medicine, drugs now are medically effective if the effect is specific: killing bacteria, relieving low blood pressure, pain relief, etc. But medicine is not entirely subsumed by the natural-scientific context. Natural sciences are more general than concrete applications such as those of medicine. Medicine embraces more than natural-science notions, such as the experience derived from a practice of diagnostics and therapy. For relating both contextures – natural sciences and a medical-therapeutic approach – *pharmaceutics* evolved as a kind of 'intermediary' discipline. Pharmaceutics is a distinct context in so far as it treats a specific problem, as something both medically effective and safe to apply. This problem is neither merely scientific (science is not interested in the application) nor only medical (medicine is not interested in the distinction of things). But this problem draws on both contexts: the pharmaceutical context is a special case as it treats a specific problem by referring contexts to each other. It becomes neither the one nor the other but remains distinct in the definitions that are produced.

In this somewhat strange pharmaceutical contexture, it is decided whether a drug is effective both in the understanding of natural sciences and in the understanding of an applied medical treatment. A placebo, a traditional herbal tea or a 'health' product such as vitamin pills are *not* medically effective drugs in this context. If they *nevertheless* prove to have medically relevant effects – such as in the case of placebos – it provokes some irritation, where the attribution to be medically effective or non-effective was correct. It is this irritability that hints at both the self-reference of the individual contexts and the links between them.

The legal contact has a paradoxical effect on the *constitution of expectations* regarding drugs. In its specific legal definition, drugs are defined as such means that are *destined* to be drugs. The question of how the effectiveness of a drug is developed thus becomes intertwined with the question of a drug's purpose. Active substances as defined in natural scientific terms are used for different purposes. An active substance originally developed for a medical application can also help increase athletic skills, heal sick animals or clean certain kinds of materials – and the other way round. The use of an active substance for a certain purpose becomes an important characteristic of the drug itself.

From an ontological entity, the now polycontexturally configured drug becomes a construction that is dependent on the coherent interaction between different contextures: medically applicable active substance + technically enabled drug format + destination for a medical purpose + corresponding packaging, labelling and bringing it to market. Such coherence, if attained, does not alter the fact that a drug can consciously or unconsciously be applied for another purpose than it is destined for or that such wrong applications may accidentally open the way for new possible applications or labelling obligations.

As a semantic form of meaning, the drug coordinates different contexts – both on a semantic and on an institutional level. Something can only be treated as a drug (at least with the financial support of health insurers) if the natural sciences, technology, law and medical treatment work together. In this case, the result is a coherent, polycontextural drug. If it does not (because the active substance does not have the intended effects in medical treatment or because legal requirements are not fulfilled, etc.), the joint reference to the 'thing' drug results in self-irritations of the participating contextures.

Inconsistent constructions: drugs, placebos and (new) magic potions

With our two concepts of modern society as functionally differentiated and of drugs as structural identities, we were able in the last section to show how the notion of drugs changed with the development of society. While drugs were framed ontologically for a long time, they are now framed in a poly-contexturality of independent contexts such as science, law and medicine. Successfully attributing something as a drug depends on the consistent inter-action of these in the first step of independent constructions. We can go now a step further in our analysis. Modern society offers a number of cases in which things resemble drugs but are not attributed as such. Placebos, func-tional food and lifestyle drugs belong to this disputed area. In this section I will make the concept of polycontextural drugs useful by analysing such cases that, at the same time, shed light on the question of what and how is excluded by a certain definition of drug.

To which degree the attribution of something as a drug is dependent on the successful coordination of the constructions in different contexts becomes obvious in those cases in which the polyphony of contextures does not lead to the attribution of a drug but to the attribution of a lifestyle drug, mere food or even a placebo without any effectiveness at all.

Beyond their historical development, pharmaca are characterised by the fact that they are credited on the one hand with extraordinary effectiveness, and, on the other hand, a lay person cannot judge their effectiveness. The two main expectations that distinguish the drug from other things are their obscurity and that the wider public cannot judge them. The condition for the application of such an extraordinary and obscure drug, therefore, is how they are embedded in contexts that make plausible not only their effective-ness but their safety as well. Something can only be seen as safe and extra-ordinarily effective if a lay person can be sure that the thing really is what it is supposed to be and is available in the appropriate quality.

For the case of drugs, that implies that their contextual embeddedness must make three issues plausible: their effectiveness, their specific medical effectiveness and their safety.

As demonstrated in the last paragraph, the materiality of drugs until the beginning of modern times was derived from the context of the medical-philosophical notion of a balanced cosmos. This context produced several distinctions at the same time. The first two drug-related properties were in particular taken together. In a medical-philosophical framing, effectiveness and medical effectiveness are the same. Remedies for non-medical purposes – such as abortion, love, eternal youth or superhuman strength potions – are excluded from the field of drugs. Such distinctions are reinforced by the corresponding social structural roles of the doctor and the pharmacist. The expectation that the drug is safe is reasonable because the doctor is expected to choose the correct remedy and the pharmacist is obliged to produce and procure exactly what the doctor prescribes. Both roles are restabilised by controlling both professional and administrative structures, which obliges the pharmacist to provide reliable and high-quality drugs. Since both the doctor and the pharmacist have to fulfil certain medical obligations, this guarantee of quality and identity exists only for medical drugs. Love potions and other 'magic' items are not available. Not least, the negative connotation of 'quackery' and 'witchcraft potions' suggests that the distinction of medical drugs as the only reliable remedies with extraordinary effectiveness was pushed through, at least on the institutionalised level.

This necessary connection between attribution of effectiveness, medical effectiveness and safety due to the medical context and its social structural backing disappears in the shift to a functionally differentiated society. Only now polycontexturality of independent contextures comes up, resulting in consequences for the recognition of drugs. The persistence of drugs under polycontextural conditions is dependent on the successful coordination of natural scientific, technical, medical, political and legal constructions of the drug. But, in contrast to the normative-medical drug distinction in pre-modern times, this coordination is no longer necessary but leaves room for interpretation. The three characteristics of the specific effectiveness of drugs, the specific medical effectiveness and their safety are now produced in different contextures.

The attribution of extraordinary effectiveness in modernity is derived from the natural scientific context. The effectiveness of a thing is no longer linked to a defined purpose as derived from its position in the general cosmos. Effectiveness is understood in the terms of an active substance, which is described independently from a concrete object, synthetically produced and modifiable beyond nature. This implies that an initially neutral active substance can turn effective for quite different purposes. The medical application is only one of many, ranging from agriculture to the manufacturing of plastics to weapons. This decoupling of effectiveness and medical effectiveness requires coordination between a natural scientific meaning contexture and the medical contexture – and it produces room for interpretation, in which coordination appears as possible but is not yet produced by contexture-specific means (like further research or therapeutic success).

Decoupling of the scientific foundation of effectiveness and the medical-therapeutical foundation of effectiveness is reinforced by the circumstance that the security of the drug can no longer be made plausible by the medical context itself. The identity and quality of the drug is mainly guaranteed by the legal context, and a lay person can identify it by the label. The requirement of official authorisation – and of quality and clear labelling – is not only the case for a drug but also applies to all manner of other things.

Medical drugs are no longer in a class of their own when it comes to safety. Instead, there are more and more things that claim for themselves an extraordinary effectiveness and safety by associating the scientific and legal contexture, but that do not claim a medical purpose. This is true not only for means far from medicine such as herbicides and insecticides, but also for such purposes from which medicine tried to keep a distance for centuries: means of increasing strength, making people younger, ending pregnancies, etc. Such products are no longer disqualified as 'quackery' but are offered in an almost euphemistic way as 'lifestyle products'.

From this example of drugs and the dissolution of a purely medical drug into a variety of extraordinary, secure but necessarily medical things, we can take away the conclusion for the societal-theory concept of polycontexturality and contextures that one can observe not only the multiplicity of contextures but also their connection. In the shift to modernity, the semantics, individuals and things are deprived of their fixed place in an balanced cosmos and given all the possibilities and risks of associations. The actor network theory offers a possibility with the concept of chains of associations of human and non-human actants, to follow the now possible linkages, dissolutions and relinkages of changing allies in modern times (Belliger and Krieger 2006). The concept of polycontexturality offers the potential to follow such linking and dissolving dynamics on a socio-theoretical level by paying attention to the mechanisms of the interplay of contextures.

Further implications: drugs and organisation

To complete our analysis of drugs in modern society, the relationship between the development of drugs and organisation must of course be considered. In the past two paragraphs I have shown that the understanding of drugs changes with the development of society. Drugs in modern society are polycontextural, characterised by the consistent attribution of a thing as drug from a variety of perspectives. At the same time, a variety of organisations participate in the development and production of drugs. The concept of polyphonic drugs may help to shed light on both the role of organisations in the social definition of drugs and on disputes within organisations themselves when drugs are concerned.

Organisations are specific to the functionally differentiated society. It may be contested whether medieval cloisters could already be considered as inward-looking organisations, or, due to the inclusive type of membership, should rather be thought of as institutions. In any terms, the polycontextural organisation, which is oriented towards several different contextures, only develops with the differentiation of these societal contextures themselves.

Because this chapter analyses drugs in modern society, the question about the relationship of drugs and organisation is restricted to the constellation under the condition of functional differentiation. Nevertheless, we shall in a moment look into the social structural embeddedness of the drug before functional differentiation. For this situation, the organisation is not relevant but rather a specific role-relationship is relevant. Like the expectations regarding the identity of drugs is crucially derived from the medical context, the social-structural stabilisation of these expectations is stabilised by their relation to the role of the pharmacist. Expectations regarding drugs count as fulfilled if a pharmacist personally hands over the drug. The role of the pharmacist is equally monocontextural as the drug in this period as they serve as a reliable identifier of the drug and they are assured of employment in the medical field.

These considerations point to a specific *independence* of the polycontextural drug. Different to the drugs bought from pharmacists in the early nineteenth century, today's drugs have nothing to do with the specific way of delivering them. The packaging, the trademark and the instructions allow the drug to speak for itself. Pharmacists are no longer needed to identify the drug, and, thanks to the instructions, one can even sometime dispense with the doctor, since the drug's effectiveness, side effects and instructions are provided. Furthermore, as a tablet, the ready-made-drug is not only decoupled temporally because it keeps longer; as a packaged ready-made drug, it also is socially decoupled. Accordingly, the polycontextural drug is primarily defined in its factual dimension, that is, the successful polycontextural definition as a drug.

This at first independent, polycontextural drug, nevertheless, is dependent on *organisation*. A legal context can impose certain properties on a thing that wants to be a drug, but to enforce the fulfilment of such requirements in the real case (and make these properties expectable), a sanctionable address is required. Since drugs are defined as non-meaningful in a first step, the drug as a thing must be discarded. Instead, the packaging enables a relationship between the concrete drug and a social – meaningful – address. As such a sanctionable address, the role of the pharmacist is one possibility even today: the name of the pharmacy and day of manufacture are in that case to be noted on the packaging of the drug. But it is equally easy in the age of ready-made drugs to create a relation to an *organisation* as a sanctionable social address. The fact that the registered name of the drug and the name of the producer are printed makes the ready-to-use drug socially adressable.

Other than in regards to the role of the pharmacist, drug companies are neither solely nor even primarily related to the medical contexture. Quite the contrary. Pharmaceutical organisations are nearly typical examples for what Niels Akerstrøm described as a polyphonic organisation: the primary purpose of pharmaceutical companies is of a medical nature as well as profit-oriented and thus to an economic contexture. Of course, as for any organisation, there are other contextures involved, such as the legal context, the educational context or, depending on the production site, even a religious context. But, regarding the primary purpose of the organisation, the pharmaceutical (both of a scientific and medical nature) and the economic context are key. This can be observed, for instance, in the manner in which one semantic is put forward against the other: the pharmaceutical industry is criticised for not just taking a medical approach to its research, for tests neglected for reasons of cost or for dealing with other people's illnesses. In any decision regarding research, costs, or investments, even in terms of staff and site decisions, these orientations potentially conflict with each other.

The polycontextural drug, therefore, is linked to the polycontextural organisation. And this is not all: beyond the pharmaceutical producer, a couple more mono- and polycontextural organisations participate in developing concrete drugs. Along the distribution line, these are pharmaceutical wholesalers, pharmacists and logistics companies; along the contextures, these are national and international medical-oversight bodies, research institutions, hospitals and doctors' practices – not to mention the courts and parliaments, all of which participate the drug-development process.

There are two closing remarks resulting from the analysis of this constellation. It is already implemented in the polycontexturality of a drug that its diverse contextures may be focused differently. Manufacturers, wholesalers and pharmacists can sell drugs either in a medical or an economic contexture. The form of the drug is only shifted by a change in the orientation, but it does not dissolve. What a drug 'is', which expectations one has of the drug, changes in its composition and the weight of the contextures involved in the construction. How the weight of different contextures change is the second consideration, which is not only due to the self-dynamics of the participating contextures but also due to the engagement of organisations oriented towards such constructions. If an economic contexture becomes too heavily involved, from a legal point of view, a thing may no longer count as a drug and create the need for regulation. Within certain limits, the focus of organisations may participate in the development of drugs. Therefore, for the research of polycontextural relationships, not only is relationship of different contextures within polycontextural organisations or within a polycontextural society important. Equally relevant is the dimension of things since they might give insight on irritations and transfers between semantic textures.

This perspective allows an investigation of the processes in which organisations with different contextural emphases draw the distinction between drugs and non-drugs. An example is the development of payments which are covered by health insurers in Germany. Until the 1970s, all things prescribed by a doctor were covered by the health insurance – including certain food items and beauty products. Gradually, this spectrum narrowed. As a result, since 2004, only prescription drugs are covered by health insurance in Germany. The criterion of prescription for drawing the line between covered drugs and other things ended a long debate over what could be a suitable criterion for such a line. But prescription is an 'imported' criterion. The distinction between prescription drugs, drugs only sold in pharmacies, and drugs that can freely be sold elsewhere is not oriented towards their medical effectiveness (which, from a logical point of view, must be the sole reason for insurance coverage). Instead, it is the possible danger of the drug in question that decides over the restrictions put on where they are sold. The introduction of this criterion in what costs are covered by health insurance may in the extreme lead to a dangerous but medically comparatively less powerful drug being covered, while a less dangerous though medically more powerful one is not. I do not want to imply that other criteria for covering costs (such as the drug format), as discussed at the end of the twentieth century, should be applied instead of the prescription criterion. What I wanted to make clear with this point is that different contextures differ widely in their judgement of what should be considered a drug, and that such a difference may have considerable consequences in everyday life.

Perspectives on complexity

This chapter proposed a way to analyse drugs in modern society. It started by conceptualising society as functionally differentiated and by conceptualising drugs as structural identities. These two starting points were put together to analyse drugs in modern society in three steps: the changed conception of drugs in a functionally differentiated society; placebos or functional food as inconsistent constructions; and the relationship between polycontextural drugs and organisation. The chapter tried to make clear how different contextures participate in the construction of expectations regarding drugs and how they interact with each other. It was made clear how drugs under the condition of polycontexturality can simultaneously be independent of specific interactions and dependent on polycontextural organisations.

In this final section, I would like to suggest potential consequences of this viewpoint. A core idea of Luhmann's theory of society is that it can produce and treat a higher level of inner complexity under condition of differentiated functional systems than was possible under the condition of stratification (Luhmann 1999, 2005c). This idea directly implies the question of how society as a whole can deal with the higher level of complexity within the functional systems. This question is all the more important since systems theory is not the only theory that suggests an internal dynamic of the expansion of functional systems. Science and economics are generally supposed to be a driving force in that regard (Heidenreich 2003). But the same is true also for other functional contextures: scientification, economisation, legalisation, medialisation – all these are applied and hint to crucial characteristics of modern society. But how is social order still possible under these conditions?

A core idea of systems theory is that society only allows for as much complexity as it is able to treat (Luhmann 2005a). As a prerequisite for higher internal complexity, functional systems cannot directly and in every operation be linked with each other. Nevertheless, mechanisms of coordination are important for the stability of the society. As such a coordination mechanism between functional systems, systems theory described the service relations between functional systems as well as the function of structural coupling that is performed by formal organisation. Organisations do apply a plurality of functional systems: churches pay their employees; central banks make legally binding transactions. Organisations serve as mechanisms of structural coupling as the common actualisation in organisation opens a canal of self-irritation of the concerned functional systems. An analogous situation can be observed regarding things. Despite the fact that things certainly are fundamentally different from organisations in so far as organisations are operationally closed in their decision-making process, while things are trivial in the sense of von Foerster (1993), different contextures do relate to things as much as they relate to organisations.

To include things into a research perspective of polycontexturality is not only a requirement of completeness. It is possible that in the change of social constructions a change in the social function of things is one of the decisive requirements for the success of functional differentiation: scientific knowledge becomes relevant out of science when such knowledge manifests itself in attributing new expectations to foremost well-known things; legal regulation is the result of things causing problems – and again expectations start at the thing; economisation and innovation pressure lead to 'new things'. Positive deviation (innovation) and negative deviation (risk) are manifested in things as well as absorbing measures of regulation and standardisation.

The social construction of things, the change in their construction in the shift to a polycontextural society and their possible function in the social treatment of complexity by mechanisms of structural coupling is thus a research perspective that promises insights for the theory of society, science and technology studies and, not least, research regarding innovation and risk. Research regarding things may be a hitherto rather neglected link between organisation and society with regard to questions of rationalisation and modernisation.

Notes

1 Gesa Lindemann argues that generally sociology focuses too decidedly on the social dimension, thus neglecting the question for the borders of the social which must be seen as evolutionarily contingent (Lindemann 2009a, 2009b).
2 An exception are modern science studies: the strong programme (Bloor 1976) as well as the laboratory studies (Latour and Woolgar 1986, Knorr Cetina 2002) show that the so-called hard reality (with a logic of two values capturable things) is formed by social (three-valued) circumstances. With Fleck (1980), Kuhn (1973) and Feyerabend (1976, 1983), the idea of a mutual influence between forms of knowledge and social structure is also applied to topics outside the realm of meaning. Still true is the Weberian word that sociology has to accept certain natural-scientific descriptions (Weber 1921/1984: 22 ff., 30 ff.). Nevertheless, the new science studies have produced enough empirical reasons that it is worth the effort to research to the social conditions of the production of natural scientific descriptions regarding this realm outside social meaning (Latour and Woolgar 1986; Knorr Cetina 2002). Unfortunately, science studies in the aftermath of Latour strive to develop a new discipline out of an empirical-ethnomethodological research programme and not to connect itself to existing sociological theory. As a critique, see Lindemann 2008).

References

Abraham, J. (2008) 'Sociology of Pharmaceuticals Development and Regulation: A Realist Empirical Research Programme', *Sociology of Health and Illness*, 30 (6): 869–85.
——(2010) 'Pharmaceuticalization of Society in Context: Theoretical, Empirical and Health Dimensions', *Sociology*, 44 (4): 603–22.
Belliger, A. and D. Krieger (eds.) (2006) *ANThology. Ein einführendes Handbuch zur Akteur-Netzwerk-Theorie*. Bielefeld: transcript.

Bloor, D. (1976) 'The Strong Programme in the Sociology of Knowledge', in D. Bloor (ed.), *Knowledge and Social Imagery*, London and New York: Routledge, pp.1–19.

Bora, A. (2009) ‚Innovationsregulierung als Wissensregulierung', in M. Eifert and W. Hoffmann-Riem (eds.), *Innovationsfördernde Regulierung*, Berlin: Duncker & Humblot, pp.23–46.

Feyerabend, P. (1976, 1983) *Wider den Methodenzwang*, Frankfurt: Suhrkamp.

Fleck, L. (1980) *Entstehung und Entwicklung einer wissenschaftlichen Tatsache: Einführung in die Lehre vom Denkstil und Denkkollektiv*, Frankfurt: Suhrkamp.

Foerster, H. v. (1993) *Wissen und Gewissen: Versuch einer Brücke*, Frankfurt: Suhrkamp.

Friedrich, V., A. Hehn and R. Rosenbrock (1977) *Neunmal teurer als Gold. Die Arzneimittelversorgung in der Bundesrepublik*, Reinbeck bei Hamburg: Rowohlt Taschenbuch Verlag.

Hacking, I. (1983) *Representing and Intervening*, Cambridge: Cambrdige University Press.

Heidenreich, M. (2003) 'Die Debatte um die Wissensgesellschaft', in S. Böschen and I. Schulz-Schaeffer (eds.), *Wissenschaft in der Wissensgesellschaft*, Opladen: Westdeutscher Verlag, pp. 25–51.

Henkel, A. (2011) *Soziologie des Pharmazeutischen* (Baden-Baden: Nomos).

——(2012) 'Soziologie des Pharmazeutischen', *Zeitschrift für Soziologie*, 41 (2): 126–41.

——(2013) 'Geneaology of the Pharmacon: New Conditions for the Social Management of the Extraordinary', *Management and Organisational History*, 8 (3): 262–76.

Knorr Cetina, K. (2002) *Die Fabrikation von Erkenntnis: Zur Anthropologie der Naturwissenschaft*, Frankfurt: Suhrkamp.

Kuhn, T. (1973) *Die Struktur wissenschaftlicher Revolutionen*, Frankfurt: Suhrkamp.

Latour, B. (1995) *Der Berliner Schlüssel*, Berlin: Akademie Verlag.

Latour, B. and S. Woolgar (1986) *Laboratory Life: The Construction of Scientific Facts*, Princeton, NJ: Princeton University Press.

Lilja, J. (1976) 'How Physicians Choose Their Drugs', *Social Science and Medicine*, 10: 363–5.

Lindemann, G. (2008) '"Allons enfants et faits de la patrie…" Über Latours Sozial- und Gesellschaftstheorie sowie seinen Beitrag zur Rettung der Welt', in G. Kneer, M. Schroer and E. Schüttpelz (eds.), *Bruno Latours Kollektive: Kontroversen zur Entgrenzung des Sozialen*, Frankfurt: Suhrkamp, pp. 339–60.

——(2009a) 'Gesellschaftliche Grenzregime und soziale Differenzierung', *Zeitschrift für Soziologie*, 38 (2): 94–112.

——(2009b) *Das Soziale von seinen Grenzen her denken*, Weilerswist: Velbrück Wissenschaft.

Luhmann, N. (1984) *Soziale Systeme*, Frankfurt: Suhrkamp.

——(1999) *Die Gesellschaft der Gesellschaft*, Frankfurt: Suhrkamp.

——(2005a) ‚Interaktion, Organisation, Gesellschaft', in N. Luhmann (ed.), *Soziologische Aufklärung*, vol. II: *Aufsätze zur Theorie der Gesellschaft*, Wiesbaden: VS Verlag für Sozialwissenschaften, pp. 9–24.

——(2005b) *Soziologische Aufklärung*, vol. VI: *Die Soziologie und der Mensch*, Wiesbaden: VS Verlag für Sozialwissenschaften.

——(2005c) ‚Weltgesellschaft', in N. Luhmann (ed.), *Soziologische Aufklärung*, vol. II, Wiesbaden: VS Verlag für Sozialwissenschaften, pp. 63–88.

Mead, H. (1967) *Mind, Self and Society from the Standpoint of a Social Behaviorist*, Chicago, Ill.: Chicago University Press.

Pickering, A. (1989) 'Living in a Material World: On Realism and Experimental Practice', in D. Gooding, T. Pinch and S. Schaffer (eds.), *The Uses of Experiment: Studies in the Natural Sciences*, Cambridge: Cambridge University Press, pp. 275–98.

Rosenbrock, R. and T. Gerlinger (2006) *Gesundheitspolitik: Eine systematische Einführung*, Bern: Verlag Hans Huber.

Schimank, U. (2007) *Theorien gesellschaftlicher Differenzierung*, Wiesbaden: VS Verlag für Sozialwissenschaften.

Schmitz, R. (1998) *Geschichte der Pharmazie*, vol. I: *Von den Anfängen bis zum Ausgang des Mittelalters*, Eschborn: Govi-Verlag.

Schulze, C. (2002) *Die pharmazeutische Fachliteratur in der Antike: Eine Einführung*, Göttingen: Duehrkohp & Radicke, Wissenschaftliche Publikation.

Schuppert, G. F. and A. Voßkuhle (2008) *Governance von und durch Wissen*, Baden-Baden: Nomos.

Vogd, W. (2010) *Gehirn und Gesellschaft*, Weilerswist: Velbrück Wissenschaft.

Weber, M. (1920/1988) *Gesammelte Aufsätze zur Religionssoziologie*, vol. I, Tübingen: Mohr Siebeck.

——(1921/1984) *Soziologische Grundbegriffe*, Tübingen: UTB/Mohr Siebeck.

2 Polycontexturality and the body

Holger Højlund and Anders la Cour

This chapter investigates how residential care homes for the elderly use various multi-observational technologies to engage with their residents' bodies. The residents' mental and physical challenges mean that residential care homes cannot rely on collecting information about the residents' physical needs and general state of well-being by simply asking them. Framed in a systemic vocabulary, they are challenged as organisational systems by the fact that the psychological systems are not able to serve as informants on the biological systems. The coupling between the residents' mental capacities and their bodily needs is no longer entirely yoked together. Consequently, residential care homes are forced to rely on a number of modern technologies to provide information about their residents' physical and mental status. Using empirical material based on on-site observations and interviews in Danish residential care homes from 2010 to 2013, this chapter demonstrates how the use of technology gives rise to multi-observational arrangements that not only allow the condition of the body to be voiced in various ways within elderly care organisations, but that also create the necessary preconditions for establishing a variety of social structures that make the residents' physical state, henceforth 'the body', relevant to the surrounding social subsystems within the organisation of residential care. The chapter's conclusion describes how the use of technology makes it possible for an otherwise silent body to be personalised and thereby connected to several function systems, thus producing a polycontextualised or polycentric body.

A theory of systems

The negation of the body is a common critique of communication theory (in general, see, e.g., Loenhoef 1997) and the system theory of the German sociologist Niklas Luhmann in particular (see Dziewas 1992; Brier 2001; Borch 2013; Borch and Højlund 2013; Phillippopoulos-Mihalopoulos 2013). At first perusal, the critique appears to be fair. The various theories, and, especially, Luhmann's system theory, seldom reflect on the body and its impact on communication. Luhmann never developed a clear definition of 'the body' in relation to communication. Comprising more than fifty books and 400 articles, Luhmann's overwhelmingly comprehensive body of work rarely ever mentions the body. Even his books on love, trust, religion and learning offer remarkably little space to the physical and biological other-side of the social. There are only a few exceptions where Luhmann discusses the status of the body. In a text on inclusion/exclusion, Luhmann observes how the inhabitants of the Brazilian favelas are reduced to silent bodies, which is marked by their total exclusion from the dominating functional systems of economy, power, law and science (Luhmann 1995b; see additional examples in Luhmann 1995a: 245).

Similar to Luhmann, other sociological studies engage in showing how different processes of exclusion depersonalise people and reduce them to nearly silent bodies with nothing to say. This is not only the case within favelas but also one of the extreme results of prisons, monasteries and camps of various kinds (Stichweh 2002; Opitz 2008). This study shows the opposite movement. Instead of analysing processes of exclusion of people reducing them to silent bodies, we show how the body exists as a pre-social entity, exterior to the social system, waiting to be included in the social system. Applying Luhmann's theory of social systems, we demonstrate how this is being done – not in the usual way, where the psychological system brings in observations that make the body a topic of a social system's communication, but through the use of various care technologies that facilitate processes of inclusion (for other similar perspectives, see Højlund 2009).

We argue that because system theory treats the body as the total exterior to social systems, situated in its environment, system theory makes it possible to investigate how the body affects the autopoiesis of social systems. The fact that Luhmann emphasises placing systems in the environment of other systems does not mean a devaluation of these systems, as some critics mistakenly assert (Luhmann 2004: 256). Instead, the differentiation between systems and their environment allow observation of how the systems make it possible to respond to operations that occur in their environment. In the case of this chapter, the mental systems and biological operations in bodies are outside the realm of the social organisation of elderly care. This chapter provides theoretical support for this argument, as well as an example of how system theory can unmask the relationship between processes of communication and the body by studying the specialised technologies of elderly care.

Luhmann's systems theory construes the world as consisting of an infinite numbers of systems: biological, psychological and social. On an operational level, these systems emerge from closed, self-referential processes, but are open with regard to observations and the processing of information. Structures are balanced in order for the systems to reproduce autopoietically. Thus, biological systems emerge from cells that reproduce cells with the help of cells. The same logic is at stake with psychological systems that produce conscience through conscience and social systems that produce communication from communication. Consequently, all systems are closed around their own specific operations. Precisely because of this closeness, the different systems have the ability to create information about the operations of other systems in their environment in order better to adapt their own operations to them.

The resulting observational openness, however, always happens on the observing system's terms. Luhmann (2012: 49–67) identifies the situations where operationally closed systems make it possible for themselves to observe operations in their environment in order to respond to them through structural coupling. Situations of this nature are visible when systems are dependent on other systems for their own development. Structural couplings allow the internal operations of the systems to be affected by operations in their environment, but only on their own systemic premises. Couplings mean the systems can react to their environment and thereby avoid ineffective self-adaptation, and ultimately destruction. Structural coupling is therefore important for mutual adaptation in otherwise closed, self-referentially operating systems. The only way social systems can be structurally coupled with biological systems is via the presence of internal observational arrangements in the form of, for example, programmes and technology that make observing the biological systems possible. In order to respond to the observed complexities, the observations are processes and turned into information (la Cour 2006).

Technologies make it possible for care organisations to be structurally coupled to the bodies of their users, which is important for the ability to take in information and process it. Each technology can be observed as related to a certain idea of causality that legitimises the use of it, in order to reduce complexity and gain a certain objective. A stool scheme, for example, functions as a technology because it makes it possible to observe when the inhabitant had their latest visit to the toilet, when they need to go to the toilet again, in order to secure the objective that they will not have problems with their digestive system. A variety of technologies can in this way be used, including observation schemes, practical handbooks and guidelines. Each of the individual technologies only exposes the bodily complexity observed to a limited extent, highlighting just a few of the operations of the body, leaving many of them unnoticed. In this respect, technologies are one-eyed. They only observe one body function at a time. As a result, the bodies seen as part of the caretaking are products of mono-observational schemes. Some aspects of the bodies are left in the dark, while others are illuminated. A fundamental premise of observational activities is that they exclude some potential matters of interest to realise others. Achieving a complete picture is impossible; the body as a whole body is inaccessible, only present in care organisations as a fata morgana or unreachable vanishing point. Obviously, this does not mean the organisations will refrain from attempting to produce complete pictures of the body. Each technology will independently aim to cover the whole, but from an individual perspective. The technologies multiply the inhabitants' individual bodies in multiple pictures, each picture representing a single totality. Each body is reproduced simultaneously as both one and many, unreachable in one catch-all picture and therefore paradoxically represented in many.

The silent body

If, on a general level, system theory has nearly erased the body from the theory, its theory of organisations, where bodies are hardly ever mentioned, appears to have done this to an even greater degree (Luhmann 1994, 2000). In systems theory, organisations represent one of the most body-free zones of society. More precisely, organisations are the decision machines of modern society, where people have roles, tasks and duties, in addition to participating in formal and informal decision-making of various kinds. The bodies of the organisation's members are often invisible to the organisation, which also appears not to take a true interest in the body. The starting point of this chapter, however, is organisations that have gradually specialised specifically in taking care of human bodies, namely residential care homes.

Historically, residential care homes have provided a home for people who, due to the biological and psychological realities of ageing, have been unable to live independently in their own homes. Whether public or private, residential care homes in Denmark are monitored by local authorities to ensure that they meet professional standards for hygiene, medication and other forms of health care. The majority of elderly residents are in a severely weakened condition, physical and mentally. An estimated two-thirds of all nursing-home residents in Denmark suffer from dementia, a rather unique illness in that cognitive degeneration generally sets in long before any physical decline. This means that individuals suffering from dementia are often physically well functioning, but are mentally and emotionally impaired to varying degrees. For obvious reasons, this puts high demands on the management and staff to create a daily life that focuses on the residents' needs and quality of life (Welfare Commission 2012).

Because people suffering from dementia are observed as having exceedingly little or no control over their bodies, the environment assumes the organisation will take over responsibility for the inhabitants' bodies. In other words, dementia is looked upon as an illness that decouples the psychological system from the biological one. The systems lose sight of each other in such a way that the psychological system only responds to extremely few biological operations and non-operations. This is the case when the elderly do not respond to the biological system's needs, for example to eat, sleep or go to the toilet. Such a decoupling makes it impossible for the intimate system, i.e. the family environment, to hold the person responsible for his or her biological well-being; instead, it becomes the responsibility of professionalised care in the setting of a residential care home to meet these needs. In other words, people with dementia do not have the necessary mental capacity to mediate between the needs of the biological system and the surrounding social system. Simple yes-no questions will not do in order to find out what the needs are: Are you hungry? Do you need to go to the toilet? Are you lonely? Such questions will not create the kind of reliable information residential homes need to deliver the expected care.

Therefore, the care organisation observes the elderly as foreigners in their own bodies, which is also why they meet them with a general mistrust. The managerial relationship between person and body is simply regarded as being out of order. Moreover, as elderly individuals can harm themselves by being active or inactive at the wrong time, residential care homes have preventive measures and structures aimed at substituting body management.

The use of technologies

Our empirical research at elderly care homes comprises various examples of technologies that substitute normal body management. For example, residents with severe dementia might be equipped with a bracelet that beeps if they suddenly wander away from their care facility, or the residential home may have electronic surveillance cameras. Another example is how residential care homes use fixed temporal structures and schemes for going to the toilet for residents unable to recognise the basic need to do so (see extended analysis in la Cour 2012). As a result, daily life is dominated by the organisation's constant control of the inhabitants' bodies using a variety of distinct technologies. The residents' lack of control is observed as a danger, which is why the organisation makes arrangements so the bodies move from being dangerous to being manageable.

In other words, residential care homes have professionalised their relation to the body, taking pride in being able to meet the body's different needs. The organisation is dependent on the use of various technologies to produce information about the body to construct an idea of the body's needs. The technologies are tools for making the body's needs visible, thus providing the body with a voice within the organisation. They also do more than this. By simultaneously organising social structures to fulfil the needs observed, the technologies make collecting, organising and memorising different aspect of the body possible.

As a result, to an extreme degree, residential care homes represent a social system where the complexity of the bodily existence and bodily behaviour challenges the way they order their internal operations. Care largely becomes a matter of having safe connections to the inhabitants. The residents' well-being means physical safety for the organisation. The opposite, a lack of well-being, is a risk to be decided upon. In structural terms, bodily well-being is a materiality continuum (Luhmann 2012: 56) for the care organisation being challenged by the ageing body itself. Even though the residential care home cannot control the autopoietic operations of the body, the system must operate with respect to the complexity of the body.

Using various kinds of technology, residential care homes as systems of communication replace the lack of information silent bodies provide. The technologies do not govern the homes, but they continually rationalise the care-giving in a manner that is not rationally planned (for empirical studies, see e.g., Berg 1996, 1998; Højlund and la Cour 2003; Berg and Harterink 2004; la Cour, 2012). At the same time, residential care homes cannot do without the technologies that make receiving information about the silent bodies possible.

As with all technologies, care technologies enhance sensitivity to disturbances (Luhmann 2012: 318). Information is taken in by the technologies in order for care to be irritated from them (for the notion of irritations, see Luhmann 1997). With a suitable number of technologies, the care is able to take in information from heterogeneous sources such as a body of cells, the psychology of the conscience and the social aspect of communication, despite the strong decoupling that exists because of dementia. In this sense, the body awaits technologies that will provide it with a voice within the organisation, even though they are always at risk of not noticing important matters. The next section presents some of the technologies that give the body a variety of voices within the organisation of residential care homes. It also further discusses how the different technologies relate to each other, how they produce different forms of individuality and collectivity and how they make various couplings between the needs of the body and the needs of the organisation possible.

Empirical findings on technologies used in residential care homes

The body is objectified and made visible through its subjection to an increasing array of technologies that lead to the identification of a variety of health risks and diseases, even when these risks remain unacknowledged by the individual. Table 2.1, below, lists some of the most important and frequently used technologies in residential homes in Denmark.

As shown, the technologies not only construct what the body needs, but they also register if and how the needs are met. In this sense, each programme makes transparent the extent to which the management has succeeded in achieving its goal of minimising the difference between observed needs and meeting those needs, although this only applies at the level of the specific programme in use. Employing manifold technologies results in a residential care home comprising many different observations that lead to decisions concerning tasks such as going to the toilet, personal hygiene, cleaning, bed-making, medication, nutrition and exercise.

The various technologies produce exceedingly different options for individualisation. Medication, bowel movements, occupational therapy and dental hygiene construct the body in an exceptionally individualised manner. For example, the body's need for medication is quite obviously individualised,

Table 2.1 Technologies used in residential care homes.

Technology programme	Delivery	Function	Voiced
Fluid intake	Amount of fluid received and when	Ensures fluid balance	Thirst, reduced mental capacity
Food	When, what and amount of food consumed	Ensures adequate intake of nutrition	Hunger
Medication	When, what and amount of medication consumed	Ensures correct intake of prescribed medication	Pain, mood changes
Urine	When and amount of urine expelled	Ensures regular urination	Urge to urinate
Dental hygiene	When teeth brushed or dentures cleaned	Ensures good dental hygiene	Blisters
Bathing	When baths occur	Ensures personal hygiene	Body odour, untidy appearance
Sleep	Records bedtimes and wake-up times	Ensures adequate rest	Sleepiness
Bowel movements	When bowel movements occur and amount of stool expelled	Prevents constipation	Urge or lack thereof to go to the toilet
Surveillance	Presence indicated	Ensures presence	Movement vs. being stationary
Occupational therapy	When, what kind and amount of exercise	Ensures exercise	Active, passive
Finances	Observes financial status	Ensures financial self-reliance	Inability to manage independently
Legal documents	Observes legal status	Ensures correct legal status	Rights and interests associated with daily living
Religious/non-religious ceremonies	Presents the body as religious upon final departure	Ensures spiritual reverence	Sacredness of the body and soul for relatives

but programmes for bowel movements and occupational therapy are flexible, creating different constructions of the individual body's needs. Even the dental-hygiene programme, for example, is designed as an individualised guide, with step-by-step procedures for dentures and preventing blisters. In this way, the technologies described construct each resident as an individual being with individual needs that require corresponding social set-ups in the organisation.

Other technologies produce limited space for individual flexibility, causing anonymity of the body as a result of being disciplined collectively to follow the routines of the organisation. If management is defined as the effort to reduce complexity, and technologies/schemes as tools for reducing complexity by minimising differences (Luhmann 1997), then management of the body represents the effort to reduce the difference between, on the one hand, the structural needs of the organisation, which means its need to create stable expectations and to build routines, and, on the other hand, the observed needs of the body made possible by the various technologies. The two sides of the difference should reflect one another in an ideal world of professionalised care. In reality, finding the right balance between the observed body (with its special needs) and the organisation's need for routine and effective resource utilisation represents a constant challenge. Every single technology creates its own challenge for the organisation in finding the correct balance between individual needs and the collective routines involved in addressing those needs.

The bowel-movement programme, for instance, represents a way to observe the residents' different needs for going to the toilet and is thus individualised. Studies also show, however, that even though this is the case, bowel-movement programmes also make it possible to adapt the basic need to go to the toilet into the routine of the organisation. In other words, the technology is being used to discipline the body's need to go to the toilet to make it fit into the daily routine of the organisation (la Cour 2012).

Sleep is another area that is subject to monitoring and observation and, as such, has similarly become a routine part of regulating and ordering the temporal and spatial dimensions of care (Williams 2005; Martin and Bartlett 2007). Martin and Bartlett (2007) critically examine how the passive body is perceived as disrupting the temporal and spatial dimensions of care, in that spending too long in bed restricts the ability to manage other aspects of personal care, such as bathing and diet. Thus, sleep/wake patterns are structured by a rational, abstract and commodified allocation of time rather than the body's inner clock, which has been shown to impact sleep patterns negatively. For example, staff anxiety about managing incontinence has been found to lead to overzealous checking, thus resulting in frequently waking residents (Kerr *et al.* 2008). The staff's changing work shifts and institutional regimes also have a direct effect on residents' sleep patterns (Luff *et al.* 2011).

Another aspect is that the different technologies, although each representing a single perspective on the body's needs and focusing on only one aspect of the body, can also be coupled to each other in the sense that what one technology makes observable has consequences for how another technology constructs needs. For instance, the medication programme affects the food programme if the body is being treated for diabetes, digestive problems or another kind of illness, resulting in adjustments concerning what and how much food the body is observed to be in need of. This is also the case with the bowel-movement programme if constipation is observed as it can affect both the food and the medication programmes.

Technologies produce their own social spaces

The technologies not only give the body certain voices within the organisation but also allow the organisation to build up various social structures around it. As a result, the technologies work simultaneously as a means for observing the body and organising social structures around it. In the organisation of the residential care homes, every technology creates a distinct social sphere for making care decisions. For instance, individual food programmes, fluid programmes and reports on well-being delimit the social structures created surrounding meals. In addition, shared programmes for mealtimes (who sits where and with whom) demarcate the sociality of eating. Other spaces (e.g., for personal care) are structured by technology programmes involving, for example, bathing, dental hygiene and bowel movements. There are many of these spaces and various couplings in residential care homes. The social structures rely on their own terms regarding who can take part in them. Both the residents and the professional caregivers are included and excluded from the many different social settings that the various kinds of technology make possible. For example, who participates in occupational therapy, who is allowed to leave the residential care home and who needs help to go to the toilet varies.

The social structures the different technologies make possible also create assorted spaces for how much the interaction between participants influences specific activities and how much the activities have to follow the routine and formalised set-up. Some of the social structures leave little or no room for the participants to develop the activity then and there, while others give them the opportunity to have a say about how the social activity should develop. For example, the technologies surrounding mealtimes produce an 'inside' in which the elderly interact and an 'outside' consisting of the regulated bodies' hunger and thirst. The technologies create a dynamic in which meals play a specific role in the interactional space between the presence of those eating together and the surrounding organisation. The people at the meal occupy an interactional space that allows the situation to define what is meaningful care for them, while outside the residential care home, organisation is a specific reference point for the inside interactional

Table 2.2 Three technologies that illustrate structured social spaces based on self-description or other descriptions.

Technology Programme	Code	Person-body coupling	Interaction-organisation coupling	Inside/outside description	Rationality/ reflexive potential
Bowel movements	Help to go to the toilet/no help	Decouples the person from the body	Situational care regulated by technological structures	Well-ordered digestion situation as the inside with bodies in hunger as the outside	Management of preventive measures in the care organisation
Occupational therapy	Physical and mental self-mastery /non-activity	Self-mastering person in a body; mental systems at risk of boredom	Self-management in situations based on pedagogical premises (as little organisation as possible)	Social space of self-activation as the inside with restless bodies/mental systems as the outside	Care through activation and care for self in managed settings
Surveillance	Present/not present	Infantilises the individual's right to decide where his or her body should be	Little room for interaction; the organisation decides when and with whom the elderly can leave the organisation	Monitored spaces as the inside with the body in risk as the outside	Care ensured due to presence of the elderly at the residential care home

meaning production. In the words of a systemic approach, the technologies frame how an interaction system is coupled to an organisation system. With regard to sub-systemic differentiation, the interaction system of the meal is distinguished by the residential care home's organisational structures, the interaction simultaneously self-referentially closed and shaped by the interactional modus and processes of eating together.

More generally, each technology demarcates a social space (often formed as an interactional room) with an inside and an outside, with more than one technology sometimes forming each demarcated space. Polycontextuality has to do with these multiple inside/outside constructions on the inside of residential care homes. From a system-theoretical perspective, polycontextuality concerns how each technology creates a specialised room for communication in order to process the elderly residents. These structured social spaces are based on the self-description/other descriptions of the technologies. In each social space, a specific social and communicative context is created with reference to what is inside and what is outside the communication. Each technology permits certain communications and observations to have relevance. The basic code of care is supplemented with second-order codes based on re-entry. The second-order codes stabilise expectations, as well as expectations about expectations. Table 2.2, below, lists three programmes that illustrate this.

Due to space limitations, it is not possible to provide an explication of all of the technologies listed in Table 2.1 and the social spaces they structure. Each technology generates its own social structure based on a code that makes managing its area possible. They also create an inside/outside based on person–body coupling and interaction–organisation coupling. This represents a polycontexuality of different self/other descriptions inside residential care homes. Each technology (and each social space) comprises rationality. The technologies have functions and are selective solely because the care-givers use them as selective mechanism. Selected from among equivalents, the technologies function by installing specific selections in the social and biological domains. If the professionals are reflexive concerning their use of technologies, their reflexivity will concern how to choose among and utilise the technologies. All of the technologies can be applied in more than one way, which represents a surplus that paves the way for a reflexive use of each technology.

The functional systems

Luhmann describes the modern society as functional differentiated. The society consists of various functional systems that observes differently and, by doing so, uphold a specific function within the society. There is the political system, which operates on the basis of establishing distinctions between who is in power and who is not; the economic system, where money circulates through the observations of payment and non-payment; the legal system, through what is legal; the care system, through what is helpful and what is not; the medicine system, which works by its differentiation of sickness and health; the pedagogical system, which observes through the lens of people progressing or not; and the religious system, by which the world is divided into believers and non-believers. In this way, modern society consists of several different functions systems that have evolved throughout history and have established themselves so that social processes in a modern society take place through political, economic, legal, care, medical, pedagogical or religious communication. People are included within these many functional systems by being addressed in communication as persons that are observed as relevant for the further communication within the particular functional system.

The point is that in contrast to organisations, which are closed in the social dimension, by their sharp distinction between who is a member and who is not, the functional systems are open for everyone. If you do not have any money, you are observed as a debtor; if you are on the wrong side of law you are observed as a criminal; and if are you without political influence you are looked upon as a person with lack of power. In other words, living in a modern society, you are evidently included within a multiplicity of functional systems. But the illness of dementia challenges the natural inclusiveness in all the functional systems of modern society. The slow but persistent process of psychological destruction challenges the person's ability to be engaged in the communication of the different functional systems, and they have for their part difficulties with constructing the person suffering from dementia as a relevant person for their communication.

The lack of psychological abilities, that is the consequences of advancing dementia, slowly deprives the persons any social definition not only within the political, economic, pedagogical and juridical but also within the normal institutions of care and medicine. This development is in danger of producing a condition where the person suffering from dementia is left without any social capital, in a condition of social nakedness. With no roles to play, at the end deprived all their dignity and humanity.

Advancing dementia is today one of the main reasons why people are becoming inhabitant of the residential homes, regardless of age. In this way, the many technologies for the residential homes can be seen as a way of preventing a total exclusion of society by making it possible for the residents to be addressed within society's different function systems. Most obviously, the technologies make it possible for the care and medication systems to approach the body as an entity in need of help and as a patient. In so doing, the technologies also connect the triad of biological, psychological and social systems by constructing the body as a person in need of help and medical care. As a result, the organisation gains the opportunity to connect to the body and organise a large variety of social structures around it. But the technologies also allow the body to appear as a person within an pedagogical system, where the person suffering from dementia is constructed as someone who should learn – for example, through the occupational therapy for exercise and dental hygiene for trouble-free teeth. The body is addressed as a person within a pedagogical function system and constructed as an entity that has to learn. There is also a programme for finances that constructs a story in which residents take care of their personal finances with their own budget, financial opportunities and limitations or in the legal system which involves technologies that produce the person with rights. Even in death, when the body is more silent than ever, there are procedures for leaving the organisation that respect the sacredness of the body and soul. In this way, the various technologies invoke the silent body, giving it the status of a person who can be approached as an individual with various needs as a patient, consumer, believer and as a citizen with certain rights. Communicative variability goes here together with technological and functional differentiation.

Seen in this picture, the technologies of the residential homes function as a way to abandon the total exclusion from the different functional systems of modern society by being included in the multifunctional social life of the residential homes. However, that would be only one part of the story. Even though the various technologies give the body a multiplicity of voices that reinclude the otherwise silent body into the communications of society, it is obvious that this rehumanisation is restricted to the resident home. In this way, the inhabitants suffering from dementia are included in an exclusionary way, because they are deprived any social contact with the surrounding world. The residential care homes are total institutions in the sense of Goffmann (1961) by creating a special zone of inclusion, complex enough to let the inhabitant have a voice within the several function systems of modern society but at the same time excluded from the rest of the society. The technologies provide the body with a chorus of voices, but they are only heard by the professional staff of the residential care homes.

Conclusion

People suffering from dementia do not have the necessary skills to take active part in communication, their ability to talk and process information (making a unity from the difference of utterance-information-understanding) as a prerequisite for a social system to occur, is not there. As shown, our assumption is that technology provides the body with a voice in the organisation where the psychological system is unable to provide enough complexity to assist the communication. As a result, the body becomes processed. In addition, it also becomes possible for the organisations to enable decisions and create social structures around the body. We also assume, however, that each technology has a certain functionality that allows only a restricted amount of complexity concerning the body to be processed. This means that only one voice is heard for each technology, which provides a particular space for information and social structures. Polycontextuality emerges as a consequence of the fact that modern residential care homes makes use of several technologies in their everyday life routines.

This chapter has primarily focused on how residential care homes attempt to relate to the body in order to be able to respond to it through observations informed by technologies. Even though it seems like a technology story, the story is really about organisations as social systems. As social systems and decision-making machines, residential care homes are multi-contextual. The dwellers comprise people with one and many bodies. In this hyper-cycle of structural couplings, residential care homes and the environment of bodies are under pressure, which, in turn, raises the issue of whether residential care homes have the requisite variety to learn fast enough from all the irritations they have themselves to thank for.

This chapter has shown how the body is represented inside the organisation as a chorus of voices that represent a challenge for the organisation to respond to properly. The answer appears to be to create numerous isolated social spaces, which construct their own forms of individuality/collectivity; needs of the body/needs of the organisation; inside/outside; interaction/organisations; and foreign/self-references. This represents a manageable challenge for handling the complexity the polycontextuality of the body represents for the organisation of elderly care. Putting internal differentiations of this nature into subsystems, however, is the residential organisation's way of adapting to the environments of the body, thus intensifying the organisation's irritability with ongoing self-irritations as potential sources of stress, because the technology increases the sensitivity of the internal social processes and constantly makes the system aware of the risk of disregarding important biological matters.

This is not to say that the technologies rule the residential care homes, but that the care homes are presupposing technologies as communicative facilitators. The social processes of care are dependent on technological back-up, so to speak. Because of the silent body of the inhabitants, the organisations presuppose technologies and rely on technologies in all present operations, because no alternatives are available. The technologies make it possible to couple completely in a structured way heterogeneous elements of biological operations with social operations without the aid of psychological operation in the psychological systems of the inhabitant. But the technologies also produce isolated social structures that exist simultaneously with other structuring elements such as the professional roles of the care-givers, general regulations coming from the welfare political system and so on and so forth. The technologies represent a complexity of their own.

In this way, it becomes a question of resonance capacity, since the system can stress itself due to all the information it makes available to itself. This means that residential care homes must be able to regulate how they can reduce the complexity the system produces. The complexity only grows when the influence the information a single technology has on how other technology produces information is taken into consideration, i.e. the turbulence one technology transfers to another. No ultimate, superior technology exists, however, that has the authority to determine how and to what degree the different technologies should relate to one another. The effects of anxiety and uncertainties challenge the capacity of residential care homes to respond to the various constructions of the body, its needs and what should be done.

The technologies present the body as a heterogeneous collection of different needs, thus making it possible to disconnect the different parts of the body and isolate the fulfilment of its needs to particular social spaces. The challenge is for the organisation to connect this disconnection by developing criteria for their mutual ordering. The criteria, perhaps hidden and shifting, for ordering the spaces that the technologies disconnect, however, are currently opaque. In other words, it becomes severely problematic for residential care homes to develop rules for how to handle the many distinctions that are at stake in its various social arrangements. If the organisation does not succeed in developing a reflexive programme that can formulate a general proposal about how the many different technologies and the social spaces they give occasion to can relate to the overall idea of the 'wholeness of care' and 'the user in focus', these otherwise sympathetic ideas will run the risk of creating the residential care home as a place haunted by its own visions about the body's needs and thus lose its ability to ensure the desired care and focus.

The result is that the body becomes multi-centric within the organisation as the body is not described in a binding way in relation to the other technologies anywhere in the organisation, thus making it harder to organise them hierarchically. On the one hand, the body and its needs are overwhelmingly present in the organisation, with nearly everything decided upon in the organisation related to the well-being of the residents' bodies. It can also be argued, on the other hand, that the body as such disappears in the polyphonic chorus of the many voices that the widespread use of technologies makes possible because the organisation does not have anywhere the body can be observed in its totality.

References

Bednarz, J. (1984) 'Functional Method and Phenomenology: The View of Niklas Luhmann', *Human Studies*, 7 (3/4): 343–62.

Berg, M. (1996) 'Practices of Reading and Writing: The Constitutive Role of the Patient Record in Medical Work', *Sociology of Health and Illness*, 18 (4): 499–524.

Berg, M. and P. Harterink (2004) 'Embodying the Patient: Records and Bodies in Early 20th-Century US Medical Practice', *Body and Society*, 10 (2–3): 13–41.

Berg, M. and A. Mol (eds.) (1998) *Differences in Medicine: Unraveling Practices, Techniques and Bodies*, Durham, NC: Duke University Press.

Borch, C. (2013) 'Spatiality, Imitation, Immunization: Luhmann and Sloterdijk on the Social', in A. la Cour and A. Philippopoulos-Mihalopoulos (ed.), *Luhmann*

Observed: Radical Theoretical Encounters, Basingstoke: Palgrave Macmillan, pp. 150–68.

Borch, C. and H. Højlund (2013) 'Critical Blind Spots: Limits to Critique in Luhmann and Foucault', *Embedded in Business, Politics and Society*, 4 (1): 64–78.

Bury, M. (1998) 'Postmodernity and Health', in G. Scambler and P. Higgs (eds.), *Modernity, Medicine and Health*, London and New York: Routledge, pp. 1–28.

Brier, S. (2001) 'Ecosemiotics and Cybersemiotics', *Sign Systems Studies*, 29 (1): 107–19.

la Cour, A. (2006) 'The Concept of Environment in System Theory', *Cybernetics and Human Knowing*, 13 (2): 41–55.

——(2012) 'Information and Other Bodily Functions: Stool Records in Danish Residential Homes', *Science Technology Human Values*, 36 (2): 244–68.

Dziewas, R. (1992) 'Der Mensch: Ein Konglomerat autopoietischer Systeme?', in W. Krawitz and M. Welker (ed.), *Kritik der Theorie sozialer Systeme*, Frankfurt: Suhrkamp, pp. 113–32.

Fuglsang, L. (2005) 'IT and Senior Citizens: Using the Internet for Empowering Active Citizenship', *Science, Technology and Human Values*, 30 (4): 468–95.

Geels, F. W. (2007) 'Feelings of Discontent and the Promise of Middle Range Theory for STS', *Science, Technology and Human Values*, 32 (6): 627–51.

Gibson, B., Gregory, J. and Robinson, P. G. (2005) 'The Intersection Between Systems Theory and Grounded Theory: The Emergence of the Grounded Observer', *Qualitative Sociology Review*, 1 (2): 3–21.

Goffman, E. (1961) *Asylums: Essays on the Social Situation of Mental Patients and Other Inmates*, Harmondsworth: Penguin.

Højlund, H. (2009) 'Hybrid Inclusion', *Journal of European Social Policy*, 19(5): 421–31.

Højlund, H. and Knudsen, M. (2012) 'Organizational Suspensions: A Desire for Interaction', in N. Å. Andersen and I. J. Sand (eds.), *Hybrid Forms of Governance: Self-suspension of Power*, Basingstoke: Palgrave, pp. 64–84.

Højlund, H. and A. la Cour (2003) 'Standards for Care and Statutory Flexibility', in T. Hernes and T. Bakken (eds.), *Autopoietic Organisation Theory*, Oslo: Abstrakt, Liber, pp. 272–95.

Johnsen, G. (2000) 'Regulering af tarmfunktionen ved obstipation, diarré og afføringskontinens', *Sygeplejersken*, 5: 9–24.

Kerr, D., H. Wilkinson and C. Cunningham (2008) *Supporting Older People in Care Homes at Night*, York: Joseph Rowntree Foundation.

Kieserling, André (2004): *Selbstbeschreibung und Fremdbeschreibung*, Frankfurt: Suhrkamp.

Loenhoff, J. (1997) 'The Negation of the Body: a Problem of Communication Theory', *Body and Society*, 3 (2): 67–82.

Luff, R., T. Ellmers, I. Eyers, E. Young and S. Arber (2011) 'Time Spent in Bed at Night by Care-Homes Residents: Choice or Compromise?', *Ageing and Society*, 31 (7): 1229–50.

Luhmann, N. (1994/1964) *Funktionen und Folgen formaler Organisation: 4 Aufl, mit einem Epilog*, Berlin: Duncker und Humblot.

——(1997) 'Limits of Steering', *Theory, Culture and Society*, 14 (1): 41–57.

——(2000) *Organisation und Entscheidung*, Opladen: Westdeutscher Verlag.

——(1995a) *Social Systems*, Palo Alto, Calif.: Stanford University Press.

——(1995b) 'Inklusion und Exklusion', *Soziologische Aufklärung 6 – Die soziologie und der Mensch*, Opladen: Westdeutscher Verlag.

——(1997) *Die Gesellschaft der Gesellschaft*, Frankfurt: Suhrkamp.

——(2004) *Einführung in die Systemtheorie*, Heidelberg: Carl-Auser-Systeme Verlag.

——(2012) *Theory of Society*, Palo Alto, Calif.: Stanford University Press.

Martin, W and H. Bartlett (2007) 'The Social Significance of Sleep for Older People with Dementia in the Context of Care', *Sociological Research Online*, 12 (5).

Michael, M. (2000) *Reconnecting Culture, Technology and Nature*, London and New York: Routledge.

Philippopoulos-Mihalopoulos, A. (2013) 'The Autopoietic Fold: Critical Autopoiesis Between Luhmann and Deleuze', in A. la Cour and A. Philippopoulos-Mihalopoulos (ed.), *Luhmann Observed: Radical Theoretical Encounters*, Basingstoke: Palgrave Macmillan.

Nassehi, A. (1997) 'Inklusion, Exklusion, Integration, Desintegration', in W. Heitmeyer (ed.), *Was hält die Gesellschaft zusammen?*, vol. II, Frankfurt: Suhrkamp.

——(2002) 'Exclusion Individuality or Individualization by Inclusion?', *Soziale Systeme*, 8 (1): 124–35.

Opitz, S. (2008) 'Die Materialität der Exklusion: Vom ausgeschlossenen Körper zum Körper des Ausgeschlossenen', *Soziale Systeme*, 14 (2): 229–53.

Stichweh, R. (2002) 'Strangers, Inclusions, and Identities', *Soziale Systeme*, 8 (1): 101–9.

Timmerman, S. and M. Berg (2003) 'The Practice of Medical Technology', *Sociology of Health and Illness*, 25 (3): 97–114.

Welfare Commission (2012) *Livskvalitet og selvbestemmelse på plejehjem: Kommission om livskvalitet og selvbestemmelse i plejebolig og plejehjem*, Silkeborg: Silkeborg Bogtryk.

Williams, S. J. (2005) *Sleep and Society: Sociological Ventures into the Unknown*, London and New York: Routledge.

Wyatt, S. and B. Balmer (2007) 'Home on the Range: What and Where Is the Middle in Science and Technology Studies?', *Science, Technology and Human Values*, 32 (6): 619–26.

Part II
Societal arrangements

3 Two ways of dealing with polycontexturality in priority-setting in Swedish health-care politics

Werner Schirmer and Dimitris Michailakis

Introduction

Background

Like other Western countries, the Swedish health-care system is experiencing severe budget problems. Among the reasons for the strained financial situation are advances in medical technology and pharmacy which enable treatment of more and more illnesses but which, as a result, give rise to more and more claims for treatment. Another obvious cost factor is demographic ageing, which increases health-care demands while shrinking the financial base created by tax and premium payers.

As a consequence, the Swedish state began to consider priority-setting in health care as an inevitable measure (Calltorp 1989, 1992, 1999; SOU (Swedish Government Official Reports) 1993, 1995, 2001). The purpose of priority-setting, it is said, is to spend scarce resources with high utility and to avoid unnecessary or doubtful treatment relative to health outcomes. Priorities are made between different medical realms, between different therapies and treatments, between different kinds of medication and especially between different (groups of) patients (Ham and Coulter 2001).

Priority-setting in health care is not just about distributing scarce resources in cost-efficient and medically rational ways; it also raises issues of inclusion, exclusion and fairness. Setting priorities 'right' is not a problem that is unique to Sweden but one common to every government in countries with publicly financed health care (Ginzberg 1990; Callahan 1995; Ham 1997; Daniels and Sabin 2002). However, the situation of Sweden is somewhat peculiar, which makes priority-setting a much more politically loaded issue than in Anglo-Saxon or Continental European political systems.[1] First, the Swedish health-care system is exclusively financed by taxes according to a solidarity principle, i.e. taxpayers contribute to health-care costs dependent on their income, but they receive health care independent from their economic spending power. There is only one national health insurance to which every registered resident is member (*Försäkringskassan*); private supplementary insurances are possible, but the exception and criticised particularly by left-wing parties. Second, according to Esping-Andersen's by-now-classic typology (1990), Sweden and the other Nordic countries are welfare states of a 'social-democratic' type, which means that the range of welfare services is much more extensive than in liberal and conservative welfare regimes. The Swedish welfare state is all-encompassing, collectivist, redistributive, compensatory and caring. There is an unofficial guiding formula *alla ska med* ('everyone onboard'), which can be described as the deeply rooted cultural self-image of the Swedish political system. Others have even called it the core of Sweden's contemporary civil religion (Socialdemokraterna 2006). This formula succinctly encapsulates values such as equality, human rights, human dignity and inclusion for everyone. Nobody should be excluded from welfare services and social benefits, regardless of age, gender, ethnicity, (dis) ability, religious views or place of residence. Because the Swedish welfare state has gained an international reputation, almost becoming a trademark with a high national utility value, any Swedish government needs to foster, maintain and protect this self-description of the welfare state (see Schirmer and Michailakis 2012: 39), especially to maintain tax morale and satisfy the voting populace.

Against this background, it is obvious why prioritisation in health care triggers problems for the integrity and credibility of the welfare state's self-description. By definition, to prioritise means to single out, to rank. A practical consequence of priority-setting is that some (groups of) people will receive treatment while others will not (or will get treatment to a lesser extent, or have it postponed). This opens up a gap between the levels of necessary political decision-making (what Weber called 'Realpolitik'), on the one hand, and the culture of equality, solidarity and inclusion in which Swedish politics is embedded, on the other. The idea of prioritisation collides with the *alla ska med* formula (Schirmer and Michailakis 2012: 40) and therefore poses a threat to the integrity and credibility of this self-description.

The contradiction between self-description and the inherent meaning of priority-setting is not the only problem the welfare state faces. Priority-setting always has taken place in the history of Swedish health care, both in macro politics and on local, clinical levels. But at the clinical level this was done by physicians' professional judgement (discretionary power). The claim for *open*, publicly documented prioritisation was one of the reasons for the first SOU report published in 1993, and it gives rise for a whole set of new problems. Given the political system's societal function of 'provid[ing] collectively binding decisions' (Luhmann 2000a: 84), and given that health care in Sweden is almost exclusively financed publicly by taxes, the welfare state is also in charge of providing a system of rules that can be used by county councils, hospital managers, administrators and physicians both in decision-making and in communication with patients and their relatives. This task is extremely challenging because such criteria must be deemed legitimate, cost-effective and efficient by all parties involved (physicians, patients, administrators, politicians and taxpayers). On the one hand, prioritisation criteria need to be 'ethical', that is, comply with the standards of modern moral semantics. Prioritisation via criteria based on ascriptive social attributes such as gender, ethnicity, age, sexual orientation and religious affiliation would be deemed unacceptable (Schirmer and Michailakis 2011: 269). On the other hand, the polycontextural structure of modern society requires a different approach to health care (Gibson and Boiko 2012: 55); it does not allow a unitary or unifying set of criteria according to which prioritisations can be made. From an economic point of view, for example, priority-setting is about saving money. Cheaper or more cost-effective treatments are preferred to expensive ones. From a medical standpoint, prioritisation is about needs and urgency of treatment, prospects of a cure, etc. From a political perspective, prioritisation is about solidarity, attribution of responsibility, fairness, coordination and reconciliation of interests. Furthermore, there are legal, scientific and religious views of how priorities should be set.

Polycontexturality means that the observational perspectives and reference problems of the different function systems involved are seldom compatible and cannot outrank each other. Medical urgency is not, *per se*, more or less important than solidarity (Schirmer and Michailakis 2011: 275). There is no 'Archimedean' standpoint in modern society from which such a ranking could be objectively made (Luhmann 1989, 1997; Nassehi 2003).

Argument of the chapter

This chapter describes how the welfare state tackles problems created by the need for setting priorities in health care – that is, reconciling the contradiction between the excluding nature of priority-setting and the integrity of the self-description as an inclusive welfare state, on the one hand – and the need for finding binding criteria for priority-setting that can be experienced as legitimate by everybody despite society's polycontextural structure, on the other hand. The chapter analyses two different proposals that have been formulated to manage these political problems. One is called the Ethical Platform; it was suggested in public investigations commissioned by the government and conducted by a 1993 Swedish Priorities Commission (SOU 1993) and updated slightly in 1995 (SOU 1995); the Swedish Parliament adopted this proposal in 1997.

The second is a proposal aimed at a substantial reform of the existing Ethical Platform put forward in a report by the Swedish National Centre for Priority Setting, Prioriteringscentrum, in 2007 (Prioriteringscentrum 2008).[2] This report is the result of an investigation commissioned by the National Board of Health after several evaluations noted that the Ethical Platform had failed in its official goal to give guidance to decision-makers and to save significant health-care resources (Riksrevisionen 2004).

As we will show in the first part of the second section, 'Two Approaches to Deal with Polycontexturality: The Ethical Platform from 1993, 1995 and 1997', the Ethical Platform reorganises society's polycontexturality into a hierarchical order with a principle on top that allows only for inclusion. This proves to be functional for the latent political goal of protecting the self-description of the Swedish welfare state, but it fails to resolve incongruities between different system-specific rationalities and consequentially to be a useful basis for priority-setting.

The second part of the second section, 'Two Approaches to Deal with Polycontexturality: Revising the Ethical Platform' presents the counterproposal advanced by Prioriteringscentrum, which, in contrast, dissolves the hierarchy of criteria and replaces it with a case-by-case evaluation which is more compatible with the polycontextural structure of society. Additionally, it introduces the idea of responsibility for one's health as a means to condition inclusion. Taken together, these measures make prioritisation technically possible without contradicting the self-description of the welfare state, albeit at the cost of lacking clear guidelines with a general scope.

In the third section, 'Consequences for Prioritisation in a Polycontextural Society', some generalisations based on the two proposals are made. We argue that the polycontextural structure of modern society does not allow prioritisation on the societal level because there is no overarching and binding meta-criterion. The proposals illustrate in two prototypical but opposing ways that some kind of hierarchy is indispensable for prioritisation. The Ethical Platform translates societal heterarchy into a *primary* hierarchy of principles in which political principles are superordinate to medical and economic ones. By contrast, Prioriteringscentrum's counterproposal incorporates societal heterarchy and thereby consigns the initial problem to the discretionary power of the physician in charge. Consequently, this makes a *secondary* hierarchy necessary. We discuss one way to achieve this secondary hierarchy, namely formal organisation. With their recursive network of decisions, formal organisations provide legitimate grounds for stratifying power and competences, thus creating space for case-by-case priority decisions. The authority of professional competence needed in health-care prioritisation – even in the egalitarian Swedish context – is based on organisation.[3]

Two approaches to deal with polycontexturality

The Ethical Platform from 1993 and 1995

When priority-setting in health care was seen as a necessary measure to handle the conflict between increasing availability of medical treatment and decreasing funds, the Swedish Minister of Health commissioned a group consisting of politicians, physicians, health ethicists and health economists to develop and propose guidelines. The result was a set of rules called the Ethical Platform, which had the goal 'to direct all prioritisations made in healthcare' (Socialstyrelsen 2006).[4]

The Ethical Platform consists of three principles. The first is called the 'human dignity principle', which states that everybody has 'equal worth and the same right regardless of their personal attributes and functions in society' (Socialstyrelsen 2006). According to the second principle, the 'needs and solidarity principle', resources should be distributed in such a way that those with more severe needs are given priority over those with less severe needs. The third principle is the 'cost-effectiveness principle', which stipulates that the ratio between costs and health benefits should be reasonable.

At first sight, the platform seems to cover different rationalities that can be subsumed in the operational logics of different function systems. In this regard, the platform responds to the polycontextural face of modern society: needs in the context of health care are matters of the medical system; cost-effectiveness refers to an economic perspective. Adherence to demands of human dignity points towards the perspective of the legal system; solidarity addresses visible collectivities and corresponds to the function of politics (Nassehi 2002; Schirmer and Hadamek 2007).

One might therefore assume that the platform is a multifaceted device to direct priorities in a variety of cases. However, this is wrong for two reasons, as we will show in the following paragraphs. First, let us look at the human-dignity principle. It proclaims that everybody is unique, everybody has the same value, and nobody should be privileged for whatever reason (SOU 1993: 95). As a consequence, it assures that nobody is excluded from health-care services due to their gender, age, ethnicity or other ascriptive category. We would argue, however, that despite – or rather because of – the nobility of these claims, the human-dignity principle does not contribute anything to resolving the reference problem of priority-setting, which by definition means *selecting* one person at the expense of another. Instead of giving decision-makers guidance in how to make the necessary rankings and selections, the human-dignity principle promotes inclusion and equality; by contrast, prioritisation inevitably requires (partial and temporary) exclusion and inequality – if not in opportunities, then certainly in outcomes. One could even note that the human-dignity principle contradicts the very idea of prioritisation, as it would imply a ranking of equals (Schirmer and Michailakis 2011: 270).

Apparently, other principles are needed to supplement the human-dignity principle,[5] and, as we argued elsewhere (Schirmer and Michailakis 2011), these other principles are actually exemptions from the human-dignity principle, i.e. criteria that are legitimate but at the same time allow for selection. This is basically true for the principles of needs and solidarity as well as of cost-effectiveness. While the human-dignity principle precludes rankings, needs and cost-effectiveness provide better grounds for this. Assuming that medical needs can be measured and compared according to suitable criteria, it may be possible to observe certain needs that are greater or more urgent than others. Assuming that cost–benefit ratios of different treatments can be calculated for the same patient groups or for treatments for different groups of diseases, some will appear more cost-effective than others. In all these cases, priorities can be set on the basis of more or less factual criteria.

However, it leads us to a problem that is directly associated with the polycontextural society: the *conditio moderna* that no contexture is more or less important than another. So, should decision-makers set priorities according to the urgency of needs? Or should they instead strive for cost-effectiveness? The official description of the Ethical Platform is quite forthright about this:

> The principles are ranked in a way that the human dignity principle takes precedence over the needs and solidarity principle, which in turn, takes precedence over the cost-effectiveness principle. This means, for instance, that serious diseases take precedence over minor ones, even though the treatment of more serious conditions costs significantly more.
>
> (Socialstyrelsen 2006)

Here we can see the *second* reason why the Ethical Platform is not a suitable tool for priority-setting. The principles of the Ethical Platform are arranged in a hierarchical order with the human-dignity principle on top. Cost-effectiveness, the only principle that explicitly has to do with saving resources, is only in a subordinate position.

Assigning the human-dignity principle a superior position has the consequence that a principle for inclusion is at the top of a platform that is actually aimed at guiding (legitimate) factual exclusion (by prioritisation). The first real criterion suitable for exclusion is a hybrid of two different operational logics, the medical and the political. As the report stresses, the goal of good health and care based on equal conditions for the whole population is an expression of solidarity (SOU 1995: 118). Furthermore, it notes that '[s]olidarity means not only equal opportunities to care but also striving for a healthcare outcome which should be as equal as possible, i.e. everyone should achieve the best possible health and life quality' (SOU 1995: 118).

Assuming that individuals do not have equal (physiological, socio-economic) preconditions/backgrounds, that different diseases strike unequally and that the curability of diseases varies accordingly, the report concludes that an equal distribution of health-care resources could increase existing health inequalities. In this regard, it becomes clear why the Priorities Commission suggests linking medical needs and solidarity together in one principle. Our analysis shows that this principle is not about priority-setting in terms of medical needs and thus does not incorporate observational modes of the medical system. Instead, it manifests a political goal of solidarity that goes beyond treatment of temporary illness but aspires to a broader scale of quality of life which is highly contingent on socio-economic status. Thus, the principle is aimed at compensating less privileged socio-economic strata.

A solidarity-based distribution related to medical needs is hence a means to even out inequalities (see SOU 1995: 118), and priorities should be set in accordance with this aim. This goal of compensating for inequalities sounds more innocent than it actually is. Taken literally, it implies that socio-economic status could be a decisive factor for what place in the queue a patient gets. The consequence would be that marginalised and economically disadvantaged groups are given priority over those who are already in a privileged social position. Not only does this, in fact, contradict the human-dignity principle, it also neutralises the medical rationality for judging needs and subordinates it to a political rationality.

Something similar can be said about the principle of cost-effectiveness. Assuming that economic criteria are important if the purpose of prioritisation is saving scarce resources and not wasting them on expensive but ineffective treatments, it is striking that this principle is ranked third and last in the Ethical Platform. The subordination to the human-dignity principle and needs/solidarity principle means another de-facto neutralisation of an important rationality.

To summarise, we can say that, at first sight, the Ethical Platform as proposed by the Priorities Commission seems to be a good response to the functionally differentiated structure of modern society by including the observational logics of many different function systems. A closer study of the platform and the arguments from the reports in the public investigation that led to it, however, leads us to conclude that the design turns out to be a smart communicative manoeuvre to neutralise medical needs and cost-effectiveness. These are the two most obvious criteria for priority-setting and thus for justifying exclusions. The logic of medical needs is neutralised by being linked to the political logic of solidarity and redistribution, which means that needs cannot be assessed without reference to socio-economic status. Even more striking, the economic logic of cost-effectiveness is ranked as least important, most subordinated and thereby rendered almost useless (Michailakis and Schirmer 2012).

As was noted by official investigations (Riksrevisionen 2004; Prioriteringscentrum 2008), the Ethical Platform apparently fails to fulfil the aim of providing guidance for decision-makers in organisational contexts who are involved in concrete prioritisation processes according to medical, economic or other criteria. In another study (Schirmer and Michailakis 2012), we argued that the Ethical Platform nonetheless fulfils a latent function for the political system, a function that accounts for its specific design. By setting a principle for inclusion on top and neutralising the two most explicit foundations of exclusion, the political system can downplay the contradiction between Sweden's self-description as an all-inclusive welfare state and the exclusionary 'nature' of priority-setting. In this regard, the Ethical Platform can be seen as a political solution to a political problem, although all of this is at the cost of the explicit purpose, i.e. providing guidance for prioritisation.

Revising the Ethical Platform (proposal by the National Centre for Priority Setting)

After practitioners and health-care administrators realised that the Ethical Platform failed to provide guidelines, the Swedish National Board of Health and Welfare (a governmental authority ancillary to the Ministry of Health and Social Affairs) commissioned the National Centre for Priority Setting, Prioriteringscentrum, to examine the reasons for this failure and to propose a new solution to the problem of how to set priorities in health care. The investigation conducted by Prioriteringscentrum resulted in a report that suggested a fundamental revision of the Ethical Platform. Among the most important changes in this proposal are a redefinition of the human-dignity principle, the introduction of the responsibility principle, the splitting of the needs and solidarity principle into two separate principles and the abolition of the hierarchical order between the principles.

Let us first look at the redefinition of the human-dignity principle. Important parts of the original human-dignity principle, such as the emphasis on equal human worth and the avoidance of discrimination on the basis of ascriptive social categorisations are again included in the revised version. The differences are to be found in the way human beings are considered:

> A general attitude among people is also advocated – respect for human worth means that we should respect human dignity. We should show respect for people's integrity. Hence, from the outset we should consider people to be capable agents who can take responsibility for their own actions. It involves showing respect by adopting a particular attitude. We should avoid, e.g., viewing people to be victims with no will of their own. A common way to avoid showing respect for someone's integrity is to 'victimise' them – e.g., to explain their situation based only on external causes.
>
> (Prioriteringscentrum 2008: 119)

As can be seen in the excerpt, human dignity is now connected to respect and agency. Respecting people means treating them as 'capable agents', i.e. beings with the capacity to make choices (Schirmer *et al.* 2012). It is deemed a sign of respect to hold people responsible for their choices and their actions. In this way, responsibility and respect become two sides of the same coin, that is, of being humans with dignity.

Opening up the human-dignity principle to agency is a key move and precondition for launching a principle of individual responsibility for one's health according to which patients can be given lower priority if their lifestyle choices (e.g., wrong diet, lack of exercise, tobacco usage) threaten their health (Michailakis and Schirmer 2010). The 1993 report of the Priorities Commission initially discussed a principle based on self-inflicted illness but in the end excluded it from the Ethical Platform. The Priorities Commission considered the main reason for rejecting such a principle to be the assumption that unhealthy lifestyles are overrepresented in lower social classes (who are said to have less education, fewer resources for changing their lifestyles, unhealthier jobs, etc.). Prioritisation on the basis of lifestyle would therefore increase prevailing class differences and conflict with the (original) human-dignity principle (SOU 1995: 26). This reasoning indicates that the Priorities Commission observes health-care priority-setting with the guiding difference of equality/inequality.

Prioriteringscentrum, by contrast, observes the same matters with the guiding difference of agency/non-agency (Michailakis and Schirmer 2012), which enables them to redefine the human-dignity principle in terms of agency, which in turn allows an 'ethical' basis for a responsibility principle as a matter of respect for being human. By defining human dignity in terms of agency and linking the responsibility principle to human dignity, the responsibility principle receives legitimacy, as can be seen in the following quotation.

> The responsibility principle means that we should respect people by making them responsible for their actions and responsible for the consequences of their actions based on individual prerequisites. [...]
> [This] is a consequence of the human dignity principle as formulated. This principle asserts that we should respect people by considering them to be free and capable individuals who can take responsibility for their own, and to some extent for other's, life and the consequences of their actions, with consideration to individual prerequisites.
>
> (Prioriteringscentrum 2008: 142)

It is precisely the attributed capability to choose that socially constitutes human beings as agents (Luhmann 1995; Fuchs 2001). Agency can therefore be expressed in obligations to take care of one's health as well as in one's choices regarding lifestyle, risk-taking, vaccinations and following the advice of health-care personnel (Prioriteringscentrum 2008: 147). Because people can choose, they can be held responsible for their actions and decisions. According to Prioriteringscentrum, these actions and decisions can be used as criteria for priority-setting:

> In a resource distribution context, the responsibility principle means that needs arising from neglecting one's responsibilities can be given lower priority in relation to other needs when resources are scarce. However, applying this principle requires satisfying several conditions, which we seldom find to be the case.
>
> (Prioriteringscentrum 2008: IV)

Patients can be given lower priority in queues if their unhealthy lifestyle can unequivocally be linked to the cause of their illness or if it has detrimental effects on the success of a treatment. The disclaimer at the end of the excerpt suggests that the main purpose of the responsibility principle is not to facilitate decision-making but to accomodate the human-dignity principle to exclusion, by making inclusion conditional on the right choices, in this case the right lifestyles (Schirmer and Michailakis 2012: 45).

The next important revision of the platform proposed by Prioriteringscentrum is the splitting of the needs and solidarity principle into two separate principles. We argued in the previous section that their linking is in fact a neutralisation of medical rationality, tying it to a political logic. The separation gives medical rationality back its autonomy and therefore provides decision-makers with the opportunity to use medical reasons for priority-setting. At first sight, the separation might also be a promotion of solidarity towards an autonomous principle. However, this is not the case. Solidarity is defined similarly in both reports as the better-off standing up for the weak. The difference between the reports is the definition of the alleged weak. In line with the observational mode of equality/inequality, the documents accompanying the Ethical Platform considered mainly marginalised people, people with low socio-economic status and those unable to communicate their needs (such as children, mentally ill and dementia patients) as the weak. Prioriteringscentrum's report strips the accompanying text for the new solidarity principle from most references to socio-economic inequality, and the only ones remaining in the group of the weak are indeed the ones unable to make their claims heard – in other terms, those who are non-agents. The connection to agency is again obvious in another statement, which shifts the meaning of solidarity from benefit to duty by linking the idea of solidarity to the idea of responsibility:

> The principle of self-responsibility is based in part on the human dignity principle and in part on the idea of solidarity among people. The former indicates, as mentioned earlier, that we should consider people to be responsible for their actions and the consequences of their actions – including their health. The idea of solidarity includes a requirement to be generally careful with public resources. Those who waste common resources subject others to problems when resource supply becomes insufficient.
>
> (Prioriteringscentrum 2008: 145)

The most important change in the revised version of the Ethical Platform is the abolition of the hierarchy of principles. The human-dignity principle remains on a separate level but has been conditioned in terms of patient agency and therefore scarcely hampers exclusionary decision-making. All the other principles, however, are now on the same level. Cost-effectiveness now has the same 'ethical' status as solidarity, needs and responsibility. This design emancipates medical and economic rationalities from the (latent) political goal of protecting the integrity of the self-description of the all-inclusive welfare state against the threat of exclusion by prioritisation and the demand to avoid socio-economic inequalities as an outcome of distributing scarce health-care resources. Putting all exclusionary principles on the same level creates a heterarchy of rationalities which corresponds with the polycontextual structure of modern society: medical needs are neither more nor less important than cost–benefit ratios or political solidarity between stronger and weaker parts of the population. Prioriteringscentrum highlights so-called *prima facie* principles:

> *Prima facie* status means, however, that one can circumvent the ethical principle without overstepping an ethics boundary – but only for

a strong reason. The most common type of strong reason is when one principle gives way to another that is considered to be more important in the situation. We find such a situation, for instance, when the needs principle conflicts with the cost-effectiveness principle. The principle that should give way is not predetermined, but decisions must be made from case to case.

(Prioriteringscentrum 2008: 109f)

'If they are in conflict, they must be balanced by ranking them from case to case. In a situation where two are in conflict, decision-makers must decide which of the principles should take precedence in that particular situation' (Prioriteringscentrum 2008: 152).

The case-by-case approach concedes a high degree of flexibility to hospital physicians, and, indeed, we can imagine very different types of cases that require different kinds of reasoning. The downside to this approach is that, in the absence of a clear order of principles to follow, decision-makers are left to their own judgement on how rankings and selections have to be made. Not only are physicians now forced to take over the task of ranking according to criteria that are based outside their natural area of competence medicine, namely on costs, solidarity or attributing agency (see Butler 1999; Schirmer and Michailakis 2011: 278). In the absence of a guiding rule-system that could be applied in a bureaucratic manner, physicians as de-facto decision-makers are turned instead into *agents* themselves; it is now them personally (and no more the system) that can potentially be held responsible for their decisions (or failure to act).

In contrast to the original Ethical Platform, the proposal of Prioriteringscentrum makes prioritisation technically possible by highlighting that prioritisation implies actual exclusion from treatment for some people. This is a merit of the reformulated human-dignity principle and the introduction of the responsibility principle. The splitting of the needs/solidarity principle and the abolition of the hierarchical order give the platform a design that seems more appropriate in a polycontextural society. As for decision-making, however, the renewed platform is rather weak because it does not provide guidance but leaves decisions to the decision-maker on a case-by-case basis.

Consequences for prioritisation in a polycontextural society

What can be learnt from the above analysis of two approaches to health-care priority-setting in a polycontextural society? We argue that the approaches are two prototypical, albeit opposing ways of handling polycontexturality. The first overrides the heterarchy of functional logics and replaces it with a hierarchical order in favour of a single function system; the second incorporates heterarchy into the design of the Ethical Platform, leaving no room for the prevalence of the logic of one function system.

We have argued that the initial Ethical Platform is a political document; it provides a political solution to a political problem. As we explained, this problem is the potential threat that prioritisation poses to the self-description of the Swedish welfare state. The contradiction between selection and exclusion, on the one hand, and equality and inclusion, on the other, needs to be blurred. This contradiction points at the differentiation of two levels of politics that require integration: the level of concrete political decision-making and the level of the political culture in which these decisions are taken. For understandable reasons, the Swedish welfare state cannot simply allow prioritisation in economic or medical terms alone. That would bluntly contradict both the cultural self-image of Swedish politics and the image foreign observers have on Sweden. Prioritisation in line with the self-description of the welfare state requires human dignity and solidarity, as they address the political *Gemeinschaft*, a visible collectivity that sticks together. Accordingly, the multiplicity of observational perspectives and function-specific rationalities offered by a polycontextural society is subsumed under the solution of this (latent) problem for the political system. It is precisely the rationalities of those other function systems (in particular the systems of economy and medicine) which could actually harm this cultural self-image of politics that are neutralised and subordinated to a political rationality.

Based on the case presented above, which is steered by the functional necessities of the self-description of the Swedish welfare state, we can generalise towards the thesis that one way to deal with polycontexturality is to sabotage or override it. In other words, prioritisation in a polycontextural society can take place by prioritising the perspective of one function system over all the others. From the perspective of any such function system, the function of that system takes precedence over the functions of all other systems (Luhmann 1997: 747).

The empirical case we observed puts the political system in the centre and at the top of society. Likewise, we can imagine an economic contexture taking the lead, which would base priorities on cost–benefit ratios while solidarity and medical necessities would be subordinated. Or, as was noted as a reason for the need for an ethical platform in the first place (SOU 1993), physicians are said to prioritise mostly according to medical perspectives while neglecting financial or political aspects.

The reformulation proposed by Prioriteringscentrum does not neglect any of the essential perspectives. The design of this proposal corresponds to the heterarchical order of society, giving each principle (with the exception of the human-dignity principle) the same status. But together with the heterarchy they import a follow-up problem. Polycontexturality means that, by default, the different rationalities, be they political, economic, medical or otherwise, cannot be brought into unison. At best, they do not contradict each other in individual decision situations; a ranking of patients or treatments from an economic standpoint might come to the same conclusion as a ranking based solely on medical criteria. Most likely, different standpoints suggest different rankings, and then one of them has to be given precedence. How then, we might wonder, can a physician decide whether or when the needs principle or cost-effectiveness is more important in an individual case if there are no criteria of a higher order that can play referee?

In our view, if one discards sheer arbitrariness, this can only be accomplished by introducing a *secondary hierarchy*. Since a primary hierarchy between the different rationalities is *prima facie* not given, and a hierarchical order of principles is rejected, another way is needed to equip decision-makers with legitimate power to perform rankings. In the remainder of this section, we discuss one way to overcome this problem, namely *formal organisation*.[6]

Although most organisations are somehow affiliated with a specific function system (banks and the economy; states and politics; universities and science; churches and religion; courts and law, etc.), they cannot be associated solely with this one function system. It is rather obvious that a hospital is an organisation in the context of the function system of medicine; however, it cannot survive by only following medical rationality. Ostensibly, it also needs to deal with economic, legal and political rationalities. If hospitals, at the same time, are operative parts of universities or research institutions, scientific rationalities then also play an important role. Hence, organisations need to be open to the polycontextural structure of society and adjust their internal structure accordingly (for instance, by having accounting departments, research departments, legal departments, etc.).

In the context of prioritisation in health care, this only aggravates the basic problem of how to combine these different and (at least partially) incompatible logics into one set of guidelines for setting priorities. However, organisations have some helpful features that other social systems lack. Organisations are the only kind of social system in modern society that allows a hierarchical internal differentiation. Indeed, they 'are able to suspend the form of equality on several levels', as was noted by Nassehi (2005: 189). The hierarchy within organisations is both the result of decision-making and a premise for decision-making. On the one hand, the whole structure of an organisation is the product of decisions in a recursive network of decisions (Luhmann 2000b), for example decisions about what positions are available and what tasks, competences and power these positions are equipped with. Furthermore, the organisational structure is the result of decisions on the relation between the different positions in terms of superiority/inferiority, coordination and cooperation. In this regard, hierarchy is the outcome of decisions, but it also is the premise for other decisions. There is necessarily an unequal distribution of hierarchical positions within the organisation. Any such position limits the (potentially free) scope of possible actions to a minimum of expectable behaviours which then, contingent on the concrete position, imply different levels of deference power and efficacy power over other positions (Collins 2000: 33), and, in consequence, over the people who populate these positions (despite the principal equality between these people outside of the organisation). Within organisations, the principal equality can be converted into legitimate inequality of the members.

This inequality is functional in terms of making, enforcing and legitimising decisions. In contrast to an Ethical Platform, which aims to do justice to a polycontextural society with a multitude of competing rationalities at play while at the same time lacking an enforcement apparatus to implement binding decisions, an organisation with its formalised rules and recursive network of decisions as well as its hierarchical structure of positions can push through decisions; ultimately, it does not matter on what grounds the decisions are actually made. Decisions are paradoxical, and consequently arbitrary (Luhmann 2000b: 123 ff.). As the cyberneticist von Foerster noted, 'In principle, decisions are only necessary when they are intrinsically impossible' (1992: 14). The general arbitrariness cannot be resolved, but it can be overplayed by the uncertainty absorption (March and Simon 1967) of previous decisions in the recursive network of decisions. What applies for organisational decisions in general applies equally for decisions in health-care priority-setting. The whole circularity of the decision-making dilemma of priority-setting is summarised in the two excerpts from the report by Prioriteringscentrum below:

> The goal of priority-setting in health care should be based on what an authoritative decision-maker believes is the right thing to do, not on what can be implemented easily.
>
> (Prioriteringscentrum 2008: 181)

> We have proposed that the ethical principles – except for the overriding human-dignity principle – should be given the same ethical status, which means that in conflicting situations, decision-makers must use their own judgment. Hence, decision-makers – whether politicians or health-care professionals – must have the capacity and sense support from the rest of the organisation in decision-making situations.
>
> (Prioriteringscentrum 2008: 181)

Both excerpts indicate that the shift from the level of different function systems (and their competing rationalities) to a formal organisation is inevitable, but at the same time it does not solve the very problem that constituted the starting point of the original Ethical Platform (how to set priorities right). On the contrary, the problem is externalised to the 'decision-maker' with their professional competence and the formal authority provided by the organisational structure. As a consequence, the decision-maker is rendered into an *agent* (as is the patient), cast into the centre of the whole prioritisation process and burdened with increased pressure to come to reasonable decisions. And still it is unclear on *what criteria* decisions ought to be based! If prioritisation criteria are applied on a case-by-case basis, the circle is closed. For reasons of practicality, ultimately, any criterion can be used to motivate the decision whenever justification becomes necessary. *Ex post facto*, many different reasons can be given, and sometimes it is difficult to reconstruct which of them 'really' had their causal share in the production of the concrete priority decisions. These decisions might be presented as due to a similar outcome in precedence cases, due to different personalities (or leadership styles) of 'decision-makers', which is a functional fiction for the organisation (see Luhmann 2000b: 136f), due to the 'professional competence' of decision-makers (such as their expertise in medicine), due to changes in conditional programs, or due to current external pressures such as time (Luhmann 2007), political short-term interests or shifting legitimacy claims in the environment (Meyer and Rowan 1977). Finally, it is an empirical question which of these case-by-case decisions will be highlighted afterwards, and subsequently criticised, contested, appealed or overruled (see, e.g., the chapters by Vogd as well as Jansen and Poranzke in this book).

Conclusion

Priority-setting in health care is a response to the growing gap between increasing claims to medical treatment, on the one hand, and limited resources to treat people, on the other. Consequently, prioritisation means that some people will get cheaper treatment than others, some will end up further down on waiting lists, and some will even get no treatment at all. Prioritisation inevitably elicits inequality and exclusion, which are both deemed unacceptable in a welfare state such as Sweden's. It is therefore a matter of course that the criteria for how these priorities are set must be considered legitimate by the majority of the involved observers (such as physicians and other health-care personnel, politicians and administrators, and especially patients and their relatives).

Even in a welfare state, priority-setting has to take place, despite polycontexturality and the coexistence of many incompatible functional logics. On the societal level, these logics cannot outrank each other, and there is no meta-criterion according to which they can be ordered. Health care mainly operates within the logic of the function system of medicine, but scarce resources, legal constraints, political interests and moral qualms need to be considered as well. This means not only that there are always a variety of competing perspectives according to which a potential ranking between patient groups, illness groups or treatments might look different. It also implies that any priority decision is, ultimately, contingent and can be called into question as being more or less arbitrary from the viewpoint of any other functional logic.

In this chapter, we discussed two attempts to bring different operational logics into an order, and, in this regard, two approaches to deal with polycontexturality. As we argued, the first proposal, the Ethical Platform from 1993/1995, transforms polycontexurality into a politico-centric hierarchy of principles that seemingly acknowledges but actually subordinates medical and economic considerations to a political rationale. The second proposal to a revised Ethical Platform from 2007 transforms the previous hierarchy of principles into a heterarchy, which is much more in line with the polycontextural structure of society. However, this does not lead to improvements in terms of priority decision-making. Instead, this heterarchy needs to be complemented by a secondary hierarchy that allows for an ordering of criteria according to which priorities can actually be set. We have discussed formal organisation in combination with professional authority and the discretionary power it implies as one way to achieve such a secondary hierarchy. In a recursive network of decision premises and decisions, each of which is basically arbitrary in itself, it becomes difficult to predict how and why a specific decision is actually made.

Organisation is not an ultimate solution to the initial problem of how to set priorities. It is only a way to postpone, move, shift the problem, but it is precisely in this regard that organisations can deal with the primary problem. In the end, there will always be a decision. Afterwards, if and when legitimisation is demanded, many elements of the (endless) causal chain preceding the very decision could be emphasised. Ultimately it does not matter which operational logic is followed, be it medical, economic, political or otherwise. In a polycontextural society, there will always be the legitimate possibility of applying yet another observational perspective from which the concrete decision can be torpedoed.

Notes

1 This is equally true for the other Nordic welfare states: Denmark, Finland, Iceland and Norway.
2 The English translation cited here was published in 2008.
3 With the focus on the Swedish welfare state, we treat health-care prioritisation primarily as a problem for the political system. This does not exclude the possibility that other function systems (e.g., law, economy) observe health-care prioritisation in a different way, i.e. define problems/solutions in other terms. The proposals analysed were commissioned by the welfare state although they claim validity for anybody involved in health-care prioritisation (i.e. performance roles of other function systems such as physicians or economists).
4 This and the following translations from Swedish into English are our own.
5 This was in fact noted in the 1993 report of the Priorities Commission (SOU 1993: 95).
6 When we discuss organisation in the following paragraphs, we do so from an outside observer's standpoint. We do not assume the perspective of the organisation itself (i.e. the management). This also means that we do not switch *our perspective* from the level of function systems to organisations. What is switched is the *object* of observation.

References

Butler, J. (1999) 'The Modern Doctor's Dilemma: Rationing and Ethics in Healthcare', *Journal of the Royal Society of Medicine*, 92 (8): 416–21.

Callahan, D. (1995) *Setting Limits*, Washington, DC: Georgetown University Press.

Calltorp, J. (1989) 'Prioritering och beslutsprocess I sjukvårdsfrågor', Dissertation, Uppsala University.

——(1992) 'Prioritering en del av sjukvårdens framtid: De oundvikliga valen', *Nordic Journal of Psychiatry*, 46 (3): 145–8.

——(1999) 'Priority Setting in Health Policy in Sweden and a Comparison with Norway', *Health Policy*, 50 (1–2): 1–22.

Collins, R. (2000) 'Situational Stratification: A Micro-Macro Theory of Inequality', *Sociological Theory*, 18 (1): 17–43.

Daniels, N., and Sabin, J. E. (2002) *Setting Limits Fairly: Can We Learn to Share Medical Resources?* Oxford: Oxford University Press.

Esping-Andersen, G. (1990) *The Three Worlds of Welfare Capitalism*, Princeton NJ: Princeton University Press.

Fuchs, S. (2001) 'Beyond Agency', *Sociological Theory*, 19 (1): 24–40.

Gibson, B. and O. Boiko (2012) 'Luhmann's Social Systems Theory, Health and Illness', in G. Scambler (ed.), *Contemporary Theorists for Medical Sociology*, London and New York: Routledge, pp. 49–70.

Ginzberg, E. (1990) *The Medical Triangle: Physicians, Politicians and the Public*, Cambridge Mass.: Harvard University Press.

Ham, C. (1997) 'Priority Setting in Health Care: Learning from International Experience', *Health Policy*, 42 (1): 49–66.

Ham, C., and Coulter, A. (2001) 'Explicit and Implicit Rationing: Taking Responsibility and Avoiding Blame for Health Care Choices', *Journal of Health Services Research and Policy*, 6 (3): 163–9.

Luhmann, N. (1989) *Ecological Communication*, Chicago, Ill.: University of Chicago Press.

——(1995) *Social Systems*, Palo Alto, Calif.: Stanford University Press.

——(1997) *Die Gesellschaft der Gesellschaft*, Frankfurt: Suhrkamp.

——(2000a) *Die Politik der Gesellschaft*, Frankfurt: Suhrkamp.

——(2000b) *Organisation und Entscheidung*, Opladen: Westdeutscher Verlag.

——(2007) 'Die Knappheit der Zeit und die Vordringlichkeit des Befristeten', in N. Luhmann (ed.), *Politische Planung*, Wiesbaden: VS Verlag, pp. 143–64.

March, J. G. and H. A. Simon (1967) *Organizations*, New York: John Wiley.

Meyer, J. W. and B. Rowan (1977) 'Institutionalized Organizations: Formal Structure as Myth and Ceremony', *American Journal of Sociology*, 83 (2): 340–63.

Michailakis, D. and W. Schirmer (2010) 'Agents of Their Health? How the Swedish Welfare State Introduces Expectations of Individual Responsibility', *Sociology of Health and Illness*, 32 (6): 930–47.

——(2012) *Solidaritet som finansieringsform och som prioriteringsprincip*, Linköping: University of Linköping Press.

Nassehi, A. (2002) 'Politik des Staates oder Politik der Gesellschaft? Kollektivität als Problemformel des Politischen', in K.-U. Hellmann and R. Schmalz-Bruns (eds.), *Theorie der Politik: Niklas Luhmanns politische Soziologie*, Frankfurt: Suhrkamp, pp. 38–59.

——(2003) *Geschlossenheit und Offenheit: Studien zur Theorie der modernen Gesellschaft*, Frankfurt: Suhrkamp.

——(2005) 'Organizations as Decision Machines: Niklas Luhmann's Theory of Organized Social Systems', *The Sociological Review*, 53 (1): 178–91.

Prioriteringscentrum (2008) *Resolving Health Care's Difficult Choices*, Linköping: Prioriteringscentrum.

Riksrevisionen (2004) *Riktlinjer för prioriteringar inom hälso- och sjukvård: RiR 2004:9*, Stockholm: Riksdagstryckeriet.

Schirmer, W. and C. Hadamek (2007) 'Steering as Paradox: The Ambiguous Role of the Political System in Modern Society', *Cybernetics and Human Knowing*, 14 (2): 133–50.

Schirmer, W. and D. Michailakis (2011) 'The Responsibility Principle: Contradictions of Priority-Setting in Swedish Healthcare', *Acta Sociologica*, 54 (3): 267–282.

——(2012) 'The Latent Function of 'Responsibility for One's Health' in Swedish Healthcare Priority-Setting', *Health Sociology Review*, 21 (1): 36–46.

Schirmer, W., Weidenstedt, L., and Reich, W. (2012) 'Respect and Agency: An Empirical Exploration of the Definition of Respect', *Current Sociology*, 61 (1): 57–75.

Socialdemokraterna (2006) *Socialdemokraternas Valmanifest 2006–2010*, available online at http://snd.gu.se/sv/vivill/party/s/manifesto/2006 (accessed 23 June 2014).

Socialstyrelsen (2006) *Etisk plattform för prioriteringar i vården*, available online at http://www.socialstyrelsen.se/effektivitet/resursfordelningochprioriteringar/prioriteringarihalso-ochsjukvarden/etiskplattform (accessed 21 July 2014).

SOU [Swedish Government Official Reports] (1993) *SOU 1993:93 Vårdens svåra val*, Stockholm: Allmänna Förlaget.

——(1995) *SOU 1995:5 Vårdens svåra val (Del II)*, Stockholm.

——(2001) *SOU 2001:8 Prioriteringar i vården – Perspektiv för politiker, profession och medborgare. Slutrapport från Prioriteringsdelegationen*, Stockholm: Fritzes offentliga publikationer.

von Foerster, H. (1992) 'Ethics and Second-Order Cybernetics', *Cybernetics and Human Knowing*, 1 (1): 9–19.

4 Heterophony and hyper-responsibility

Niels Åkerstrøm Andersen and Hanne Knudsen

One of the current challenges facing the health system is that it depends on non-health factors as it recognises that the individual's health depends not only on nutrition and sporting activity but also on factors such as their job, family situation and level of education. This makes it difficult for the health system to take responsibility for defining what health responsibility includes. Therefore, since the late 1980s, one of the governing ambitions of the health system has been to make citizens responsible for their own situation. This tendency to call for personal responsibility also has its effect on the education system (Knudsen 2009, 2010, 2011; Knudsen and Andersen 2014) and the economic system (Nullmeyer 2006). Within a Foucauldian tradition there has been a focus on this tendency to govern with a view to achieving responsibilisation (Rose 1999), but in a systems-theoretical sociology, very little has been written about personal responsibility. Personal responsibility isn't a very obvious thing to focus on within a systems-theoretical framework. There are mainly two ways in which Niklas Luhmann discusses responsibility. The first way has to do with the creation of fictions of persons and actors. Luhmann writes about the attribution of responsibility as a mechanism for creating addresses in communication. Thematising an event as an action and attributing the responsibility for the action to a specific system constructs this system as an actor in the communication (Luhmann 1995: 165–6). This is a limited concept of responsibility restricted to attribution processes, and leaving out personal responsibility and questions about how responsibility is received. The second way responsibility is discussed in systems theory is in terms of morality. Implicitly, personal responsibility is observed as a moral question, and morality is analysed as a code with two sides: recognition (good)/misrecognition (bad). Luhmann makes us aware that the moral code is asymmetric in the sense that communicating misrecognition involves a higher connectivity than communicating recognition. Moral communication, then, has a tendency to produce conflicts where misrecognition simply produces more misrecognition, and so forth (Luhmann 1993). When responsibility is regarded as moral, Luhmann does not put a lot of hope to personal responsibility (1987). And, luckily, in his view modern functionally differentiated society depends not on personal responsibility but on impersonal roles formed by binary code systems (Stichweh 1997). So in systems theory we have good reasons not to overemphasise personal responsibility.

The challenge is that it is important to focus on personal responsibility. We think the form of personal responsibility is currently changing, and we therefore find it important to focus on this change. How do we understand this from a systems-theoretical setting? To us, it is not a satisfying solution just to say that it really does not matter because function systems are not founded on personal responsibility. Dimitris Michailakis and Werner Schirmer observe a similar shift from collective to individual responsibility for health in the Swedish welfare state and argue that 'attribution [to individuals] is a communicative steering device the political system can make use of in order to keep control over increasing claims for medical treatment' (Michailakis and Schirmer 2010: 3). We do not doubt this conclusion, but we believe that the expectation structures condensed in the expression of 'responsibility' might be trickier than presumed by Michailakis and Schirmer. It is not enough to explain personal responsibilisation in the gaze of political systems. We have to ask more generally, 'What kind of problem is the call for more personal responsibility an answer to?' And we also need to ask, 'How is personal responsibility constructed here? What is its form? And which paradoxes does it install?'

Basically, we argue that a new form of personal hyper-responsibility is the answer to a heterophonic context in which many function systems are highly dependent on each other and simultaneously available to organisations. In this chapter, the term 'heterophony' is used to describe a decision and steering situation in which the codification is not given in advance (which does not mean that all codes are equal) and where the contingency of code selections and the switching between codes is observed as an important governance resource. Heterophony is observed by the organisations as a resource of potentiality.

With the health area as our point of observation, we will argue for the following theses:

1. The health system and health organisations reflect how health depends on non-health factors. It becomes an articulated challenge how to bring in and steer non-health perspectives in order to increase health.
2. One of the solutions (the solution we are studying here) is to make the individual responsible for the bridging of health and non-health perspectives.
3. There is no simple way to add up various perspectives and then address them to individuals. What seems to be the chosen solution is instead to design a number of communicative technologies that construct 'heterophonic spaces' in which codes and perspectives are able to switch and where the steering potentiality of the individual coding is investigated

during discussions of personal responsibilities. The technologies are 'health dialogues', 'health partnerships' and 'health games'.
4.   Personal responsibility is reformulated as hyper-responsibility in order to function as a medium in these heterophonic steering technologies.

So we are not going to show that functional differentiation is 'rehumanised' or 'de-differentiated' through individuals who bring heterogeneous issues into individual personal decisions. Our story is more complex. Health recognises the need of non-health. The many perspectives are linked through technologies of dialogues, partnerships and games, but these just result in even more complexity handled through indeterminacy. Individualisation means that individuals are invited to reflect upon themselves in the gaze of the function system. But this does not bridge the systems. On the contrary, reflexivity is always reflexivity within a system, meaning that reflexivity merely deepens the gaps between the systems. New personal responsibility is expected in order to create self-steering in the image of the systems; and technologies such as dialogues, partnerships and games in which individuals are expected to demonstrate their ability and capacity to take a personal responsibility are being designed. But again this just makes it even harder for the individual to identify what it means to be responsible, and for the function system to trust responsibility, because when individuals do not know what it takes to be responsible, they become incalculable for the system. So we claim that a new form of hyper-responsibility emerges as an equivalent to heterophony. But we also demonstrate the tragedy of the movement. A solution is not found. Instead, paradoxes are pushed around.

We don't claim to come up with an empirically well-documented, fully fleshed-out theory. The chapter is more in the nature of a diagnostic essay putting pieces together in order to produce possible patterns opening new questions. In this sense, our chapter is more like a programme for pushing the governmentality discussion of the responsibilisation of individuals further by connecting it to the systems-theoretical discussion of functional differentiation and organisational heterophony. We draw on empirical material from a Danish context and give priority to empirical details and richness over the possibility to generalisation.

Addressing and suspending responsibility: A healthy call for heterophony

We start in the heterophonic ambiguity in the call of the health systems for more personal responsibility. We see a call for non-health perspectives when the health system addresses personal responsibility for health. This is at least very clear in a Danish context, where the campaign organisers, the Danish Health and Medicines Authority, define it this way: 'Central to health promotion is the notion that the individual needs to be good at mastering his or

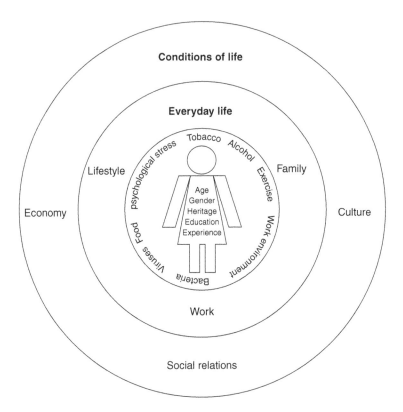

Figure 4.1 Model for health in a social context.

her life, and, as public authorities, we need to help create the best possible framework. The ability to master one's life is not always a private matter' (Danish Health and Medicines Authority 2002: 11). This means that health policy is defined as depending on other policy fields and should be a horizontal policy orchestrating other vertical policy fields: 'The Public Health Programme is meant to ensure political responsibility for an effective prioritisation and coordination of preventive efforts across sectors, administrative levels and competencies' (Ministry of Health 1999: 6; Højlund and Larsen 2001). This also makes it more difficult to delimit health problems. The Danish government's catalogue of ideas for a programme of public health illustrated the problem (see Figure 4.1).

The model indicates the difficulty of delimiting health problems. The health and well-being of the individual is perceived as a result of immediate strains on the health such as tobacco, alcohol and poor nutrition. These, in turn, are linked to particular circumstances such as family, work and lifestyle, which, in turn, are linked to more general living conditions within society: social, economic and cultural relations. Health is said to concern *lifestyle* (how we choose to live our lives, including eating and exercise habits), *living conditions* (the framework within which we are able to choose, including work and housing), *quality of life* (what makes us feel happy), *physical well-being* (feeling good about and within our bodies), *psychological well-being* (feeling good about our mental condition, including self-esteem) and *social well-being* (our ability to partake in a communal space, including making friends). This definition of health leaves no aspect of life to be defined outside the domain of health policy. Life in all its facets becomes a health concern.

This means that the health system recognises the needs of non-health perspectives. The individual should be responsible for their health, but the health system knows that enacting this responsibility depends on the educational level of the individual as well as on their work situation, family situation, culture, economy, etc. So a new problem emerges: how can the health system insist on more personal responsibility concerning health knowing that individual health as well as individual capacity to be responsible are highly complex? How can one insist on health responsibility knowing that better health might depend on suspending the focus on health issues and focusing instead on getting a job?

Here heterophony does not begin from the outside. It is the health system that invites non-health perspectives in order to help individuals to solve their health challenges.

Three steering technologies opening for hyper-responsibility

These very complex and potentially paradoxical governing ambitions call for new forms of steering technologies. We observe at least three such steering technologies through which the health system tries to create a contingent space in which an infinite number of codes can occur in a flexible way. These spaces are heterophonic in the sense that no code is privileged in advance. There are no fixed rules or structures orchestrating the codes. Of course, the technologies basically refer to health as their fundamental purpose. But they only work if the health agenda is put aside. As pointed out in relation to one of the health promotion technologies: 'Health promotion should not focus too much on health promotion.'[1]

The three types of technologies we find are: health dialogues, health partnerships and health games. They are not always distinct but are mixed in different ways in the specific technology.

Health dialogues

Health dialogues are publicly organised dialogues between public authorities and individual citizens on health issues in order to increase personal health responsibility. Health dialogues are usually highly conceptualised. In other words, their purpose, forms, rules and dialogue procedures are described, giving them a repeatable technological form, with the public authority being entitled to expect a certain process to take place and a certain horizon of possible results to be achieved if a specific dialogue concept is chosen by the health professional. Examples of health dialogue concepts are: 'The health dialogue' (Danish Medicines and Health Authority 2010: 22), 'The necessary talk', 'The motivation talk' (Danish Society for General Medicine 2001) and 'The wish cards' (Danish Medicines and Health Authority 2010: 24).

The dialogues are, in general, motivated by health issues but are designed to open up for non-health perspectives. As pointed out in one of the concepts: 'All these areas represent important elements of a healthy life and are of equal importance in the dialogue' (Danish Veterinary and Food Administration *et al.* 2007). Through the dialogues, the health professional is able to investigate the communicative potentialities in the various codes. Where is the connectivity high and where is it low? When do citizens involve themselves in health issues and when do they exclude themselves by choosing not to connect? Where does it make sense to discuss potential responsibilities without too much resistance? The Danish Ministry of Health defines the health dialogue as one 'where the citizen gets opportunities to reflect about his or her own health', becoming more aware of taking responsibility for their own lifestyle and health, and, as a part of this, accepts offers of health-promoting activities from the municipality (Danish Medicines and Health Authority 2010: 22).

The health dialogues are described by the health professional exactly as dialogues. Investigating this issue more carefully turns out not to be so simple. Basically, public law defines the relation between public professional and private citizens as a hierarchical relation where the public professional has a number of options for so-called unilateral decisions. In this gaze, health dialogues represent a unilateral call for mutual dialogue. So the difference unilateral/mutual is reentered on the unilateral side of the difference. As formulated in one of the concepts, 'Participation is obligatory because the dialogue is planned and in the programme, but people must decide themselves how much they want to be involved' (Danish Medicines and Health Authority 2010: 24). What is the function of this? It is to invite the citizen to invite the public authorities to take part in a discussion of personal matters (Knudsen 2010, 2011). Such initiatives are usually presented as if their aim is to empower individual citizens, but they also empower the public authorities by giving them access to the individual private sphere (Andersen 2007). A double-bind structure of expectations makes it possible for the public authorities to alternate between two-way dialogue and 'dialogue' pointing only to a sense of responsibility concerning their health among citizens.

The hash dialogue

The hash dialogue is a concept published in 2005 by the Danish Committee for Health Education. The concept was designed for use by professionals working with young people in various welfare institutions, and the stated purpose of the dialogue is 'to provide young people with better-informed and more flexible views on smoking hash, thereby helping them to make positive changes for themselves' (Danish Committee for Health Education, 2005: 2).

The concept emphasises that hash can be viewed in various ways and that it is vital to remember this when professionals wish to focus on it. This point is illustrated by quoting the views of two different professionals. The first of these is a prevention consultant who says 'I don't think you can use the term "treatment" in connection with hash. You can't abuse hash.' And the second is the leader of a treatment institution who says 'I view hash as a serious matter. Hash does far more damage than heroin and cocaine.' So hash can be perceived in a variety of ways, and professionals also differ as to their views on hash.

There are at least three codifications of hash in the concept:

1. a *pedagogical* codification, whose focus is to change the perceptions of young people about hash;
2. a *medical* codification, whose focus is on the impact of hash on health; and
3. a *care* codification, whose purpose is to help young people to solve their social problems – with hash being only one of these.

The concept emphasises the need to create 'an open and equal dialogue', which means that all three codifications need to be combined. The pedagogical communication should not involve instruction. The medical communication should not involve treatment. And the care communication should not be paternalistic. As stated in the description of the concept, 'It is not about treatment but about a dialogue involving mutual trust', and 'Adults must be able to discuss this issue based on precise knowledge without the system applying emotional pressure and adopting a paternalistic attitude.'

This means that the dialogue and the grounds of the dialogue must be created from within the dialogue. The dialogue aims at scanning communication possibilities. The coding depends on what creates openings in the dialogue. The concept does not take it for granted that young people will connect to the communication. So the concept does not establish simple premises for the dialogue but rather sets up ways of scanning for possible communication. In this light, the codes constitute a repertoire rather than actual premises. The dialogue offers young people room for reflection and articulation.

The concept includes various techniques for scanning communication possibilities. One of these is 'the structure of the dialogue'. This structure is drawn as two axes crossing each other, the degree of hash-smoking problems on the horizontal axis and the degree of general/specific issues on the vertical axis. The idea is that you can explore possibilities of communication with young people by alternating between talking about general knowledge about hash and the young people's own experiences. It is important to avoid statements such as 'This applies to lots of people – so it applies to you too', preferring statements such as 'This applies to lots of people – how does it seem from your point of view?' Another scanning technique starts in a figure with two circles overlapping each other, creating an intersection. One circle marks the theme of 'smoking hash', while the other marks the theme of 'problems'. This intersection is called 'the field of investigation'. The idea is that the relationship between hash and problems cannot be established before a dialogue has been conducted. It is the intersection that is subject to joint investigation and discussion, and it is important that no final conclusions are drawn before the intersection has been discussed. The dialogue investigates the possibilities for and limits to the dialogue. A third scanning technique is about inviting young people to describe their attitudes to smoking hash using a table with four boxes: advantages of continued smoking, disadvantages of continued smoking, advantages of quitting smoking and disadvantages of quitting smoking. These three techniques make it possible to keep the lines of communication open and alive, scanning them for potentialities and ensuring that the whole process of communication includes a variety of perspectives with the emphasis being placed on the development and continuation of the communication process rather than on the choice of any specific perspective.

Health partnerships

Health partnerships are second-order contracts with individual citizens or with families stating how they are expected to steer themselves. Partnerships are usually an extra brick on top of the health dialogue (for the contractualisation of the citizen, see Andersen 2004, 2007, 2008a). So you begin to build up a dialogue with citizens and end up by offering them a partnership for self-development. Examples are 'The health collaboration agreement' (based on wish cards) (Danish Medicines and Health Authority 2010: 26), 'The Yum-Yum agreement pages' (Andersen 2009, 2011) and 'The alcohol agreement' (Rasmussen and Toft 2005).

In systems theory, we can describe a contract as a form of communication that is based on the distinction between obligation and freedom. A contract is a voluntary binding of freedom. Health partnerships are a bit different. In health partnerships between health authorities and individual citizens, the contract is somehow doubled into a first- and second-order contract (Andersen 2008b). If a contract is to be observed as a promise presuming that the contractors possess the rights of freedom, then a second-order contract is a promise about future promises. Partnerships allow a certain indeterminacy to exist. To promise to promise is both to promise and not to promise. In this sense, partnerships become a technology for a flexible obligation, obliging the citizen to take health responsibility but not specifying what it means. So a partnership is a committing but not binding dialogue, an unbinding binding.

There is yet another aspect to health partnerships. The obligation which the administration seeks to form in the citizens' partnership is the citizens' obligation to reflect upon the relationship between freedom and responsibility. It is the obligation to commit oneself, to give oneself to oneself as a free person searching for responsibility (in the language of the health professional). It is an obligation to translate obligation into freedom and personal responsibility. And this is rather paradoxical.

The parental agreement on alcohol is an example of the restoration of freedom as obligation. The basic idea here is that schools encourage parents of older children to make agreements within the school class about alcohol. This agreement could contain elements such as 'No alcohol at parties', 'Adults present at all parties' or 'We will contact each other if we have worries about our children.' The school arranges the meeting at which the parents are expected to make the agreement. It is a partnership agreement because it is not only about agreeing on specific rules or obligations; it is also about agreeing to trust each other, work together and to interfere in each other's lives on these issues. The concept states that 'Discussing the way in which our children or young people spend time together does not constitute gossip about other people's children or criticism of other parents. We agree that it's OK to contact each other if we experience problems with other people's children' (Danish Medicines and Health Authority, Danish Ministry of Education, Danish National Council for Children, and Danish Committee for Health Education 2005: 9). It is stressed that some parents might choose to ignore the agreement occasionally. For instance, if they are giving a party to celebrate their child's confirmation, they may wish to serve alcohol to the young people who are there as well as to the adults – their family may have a tradition for doing this kind of thing. The concept underlines that in such circumstances the parents of other young people who are going to attend such parties should call in for a meeting to insist on their collective responsibility to comply with the agreement.

Again, the concept is designed to be flexible in order to meet the paradoxical challenges in the ambition of governing health without pointing to certain rules or norms. Governing parents' ways of handling their teenage children's use of alcohol is ambitious and takes place in a setting where alcohol is only one out of a number of possible issues on the parents' agenda. The parental agreement on alcohol handles this by letting the parents be the partners in the partnership. It is not an agreement between the school (or the health board) and the parents; it is an agreement between the parents.

Being able to oscillate between promise and non-promise, binding and non-binding obligation, the partnership becomes a technology for investigating the capacity of commitments in various codings. The immanent questions in partnerships are as follows. What is the potentiality to commitment in the code of health? What is it in the code of learning? What is it in the code of care? etc. So partnerships become a possibility machine scanning various function systems for possibilities for commitments.

Health games

Health games aim at expanding the imagination of possible health issues and personal health responsibilities. Health games aim at creating playful communication in which the individual is able to investigate the potentiality of health distinctions. Health games often work in connection with dialogues and agreements and function to increase the imagination of potential responsibilities and views in dialogues and partnerships. Examples of health games are: 'Dialogue games on alcohol' (Rasmussen and Toft 2005), 'The playful cooking book', 'Dialogue – a game on attitudes' and 'Who is the bottle pointing at?' (Andersen 2011).

Gregory Bateson suggests that play is a special form of communication in which the message is that 'these actions in which we now engage do not denote what those actions *for which they stand* would denote' (2000: 180). When children play-fight, they continually draw up a distinction between play-fighting and fighting. Thereby, they establish that a marked strike signifies the strike but does not signify that which a strike would signify. Bateson's final and more precise formulation is, 'These actions in which we now engage do not denote what would be denoted by those actions which these actions denote' (2000: 180). Thus, play represents a distinct communicative doubling machine. Play doubles the world so that we have a world of play and a real world, and the doubling takes place on the side of the play. Dirk Baecker (1999: 103) formulates it in this way:

> In play, socialness is constituted by ways of reflection onto itself as the other side of itself. In play, socialness is experienced as what it is, namely as contingent, roughly meaning that it is neither necessary nor impossible, or again, given yet changeable. Play in general reveals the form of the social by which the play infects the world.

Play represents a communicative sociality, which is characterised by its doubling of this sociality so that the contingency of the social reality becomes visible. In play, certain rules exist. Hans Georg Gadamer says that in play you forget yourself, you dedicate yourself totally to the play process (1985: 92).

A Danish campaign from 2008 organised by the Danish Ministry of Food, Agriculture and Fisheries is called 'Healthy through Play'. The campaign is designed primarily for vulnerable families and targets their willingness, knowledge and capacity in terms of living a healthy life with respect to both food and exercise. As the website says. '"Health through play" is a health-pedagogical tool'.[2] Play is articulated as the fundamental means of achieving health promotion. The campaign motto is 'to make it easy, fun, and manageable to live a healthy lifestyle'.[3] Health responsibility is presumed to be a burden which is too heavy for individual citizens to carry.

But health games are not simply play. They are administrative public game concepts, and the public invitations to citizens to take part in the games are not entirely voluntary. So, to health games, 'playfulness', 'dedication', 'forgetting yourself' and 'flow' are not simply factual events either happening or not; they are prescriptions and norms. The health game has a double-bind expectation structure commanding, 'Do as I say: be authentic by forgetting yourself in play.'

One example of a health game is called Health at Play. It is intended for use in the context of parent events, pedagogical days or events for older students in schools. It takes approximately two hours to play. The game is instructed by a teacher and is set up by dividing parents into groups. Each group has a game board with three spaces entitled 'agree', 'partially agree' and 'disagree' on the table. Each of the groups is given a stack of statements. Some of these are as follows. 'It is not okay for students to try alcohol at home', 'Parents are children's most important role models', 'Children and young people need to be motivated to live a healthy lifestyle' and 'Children and young people must learn to take responsibility for their own health.' In the first two steps of the game, the participants are encouraged to have a playful dialogue around the many statements investigating what health responsibility might be and for whom. The function of the statements is to stimulate the imagination of the participants with regard to both themes and perspectives, thereby encouraging the parents to discover new potential personal responsibilities. First, the groups discuss the statements and classify them into the statements they agree with, disagree with or partially agree with. In this way they investigate each other's basic perspectives. In the second step, the group focuses on the statement cards that the group agrees with. Three statements are prioritised and the dialogue shifts towards suggestions for actions for parents, students and the school respectively in response to the individual statements. You might say that the first step is an investigation of general norms about health responsibilities and the second step is about how you as an individual would answer the specific responsibilities in actions. So, in the second step, the participants are invited into a hypothetical game, raising questions such as 'If this is the norm for personal responsibility and this is the situation, then how would you act order to behave responsibly?'

After the first two steps, the whole dialogue shifts from game to decision. The groups now present their suggestions to each other, and the game instructor sums up the selected statements in a table of priorities,

calling it a collective agreement, which is subsequently emailed to all participants 'so that we all know which agreements have been reached'. The
instructor suggests that the collective agreements should be evaluated at
subsequent parent meetings. So here we move from a playful game to a
unilateral, organised collective partnership. The game refers to 'collective
agreements', which can be reached together with parents as if they were
one legal subject. But the parents are not a collective. So the partnership is
not really binding, or, rather, it is simultaneously binding and not binding,
just promising later commitment. And the planned evaluation at a later
parent meeting is only able to relate to the agreement as one of second
order.

Personal responsibility

Before discussing how the three types of technologies turn personal responsibility into a steering media equivalent to heterophonic conditions, we will
shortly discuss how personal responsibility in general might be conceptualised if we observe it as a particular form of communication or at least as a
semantic form distributing expectation in a certain way. This discussion will
take the form of a systems-theoretical reading of Søren Kierkegaard and
Jacques Derrida. The question is how we can conceptualise personal responsibility, and the way to answer this question goes through the question,
'What is the structure of expectation in personal responsibility?' or, more
precisely, 'What is expected of individuals to expect of themselves in order
to act in a personally responsible fashion?' We are looking for the unity
of difference structuring expectations. We ask, 'Through which distinction
does personal responsibility emerge as an expectation?'

Let's begin with Kierkegaard's observations on this point:

> Duty is the universal which is required of me; so if I am not the univer-
> sal, I am unable to perform duty. On the other hand, my duty is particu-
> lar, something for me alone, and yet it is duty and hence the universal.
> […] for I can do duty and yet not do my duty, and I can do my duty and
> yet not do duty.
>
> (Kierkegaard 1946: 221)

Kierkegaard is aware that it is not possible to fulfil the expectation
condensed in the form of personal responsibility by living up to the general expectations in one's surroundings regarding responsibility. Personal
responsibility is your own responsibility. It cannot be derived from norms,
rules and ethics. Your responsibility is only yours and should not respond
to others. Kierkegaard also makes us aware that if we expect responsibility
of others we have to trust them to be responsible by not making our expectation explicit. In his book *Either/or*, he has an example, which is presented
as autobiographical:

I knew only one duty, that I was expected to attend school, and in this respect I was left entirely to my own responsibility [...] I was exempted from all parental twaddle. My father never asked me about my lessons, never heard me recite them, never looked at my exercise book, never reminded me that now it was time to read, now time to leave off, never came to the aid of the pupil's conscience, as one sees often enough when noble-minded fathers chuck their children under the chin and say, 'You had better be doing your work.' When I wanted to go out he asked me first whether I had time. That I was to decide for myself, not he, and his query never went into details. I am perfectly certain that he was deeply concerned about what I was doing, but he never let me observe this because he wanted my soul to be matured by responsibility.

(Kierkegaard 1946: 225)

Kierkegaard's father expected his son to demonstrate a sense of personal responsibility but never fully articulated this. Nor did he announce any expectation about specific actions and decisions. Thereby, the father avoided to turn the responsibility of Kierkegaard into duty, defined from somewhere outside Kierkegaard.

Derrida pushes Kierkegaard's analysis further, saying that the possibility of responsibility begins in the impossibility of responsibility (1992: 24). *Personal responsibility* is split into two incommensurable forms that have yet to be connected: absolute responsibility, where you respond to no one and do not follow the common rules or norms; and general responsibility, with its ethics, norms and rules obliging everybody. *Absolute responsibility*, where you stand all by yourself, is an individual form of responsibility that nobody can replace. One cannot take or carry the responsibility of another. You take your decision alone, with nobody and nothing to refer to, breaking with tradition, authority, rules.

But what is also implied (in absolute responsibility) is that by not speaking to others, I don't account for my actions, that I answer for nothing [*que je ne réponde de rien*] and to no one, that I make no response to others or before others. It is both a scandal and a paradox.

(Derrida 1992: 60)

Your responsibility is not a response to any explicit demand. 'Secrecy is essential to the exercise of this absolute responsibility as sacrificial responsibility' (Derrida 1992: 67). You cannot explain your choice through a reference to general rules; it is your decision that cannot be explained: 'Hence the activating of responsibility (decision, act, *praxis*) will always take place before and beyond any theoretical or thematic determination. It will have to decide without it, independently from knowledge' (Derrida 1992: 26). *General responsibility*, on the other hand, is where you have to give an account of your actions in relation to expectations in your environment. General responsibility

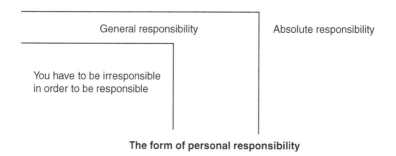

The form of personal responsibility

Figure 4.2 The form of personal responsibility.

consists of ethics, rules and norms. The two forms are incommensurable, because you can only carry absolute responsibility by rejecting your general responsibilities. Only by rejecting some expectation you show your ability to make a personal choice. Yet you have to, if you should take your personal responsibility, to take both absolute responsibility and thereby rejecting general responsibility, and to take general responsibility. So you have to take both forms of responsibility, but at the same time they exclude each other. The personal responsibility is constituted as a paradox, where one is only absolutely responsible if one is at the same time generally irresponsible. 'As soon as I enter into a relation with the other, I know that I can respond only by sacrificing ethics, that is, by sacrificing whatever obliges me to also respond, in the same way, in the same instant, to all others' (Derrida 1992: 68).

The result is a re-entry of the two concepts of responsibility on the absolute side of the distinction: You are only personally responsible if you are both absolutely and generally responsible in an absolute and singular manner. This structure of expectations can be depicted as shown in Figure 4.2.

Every concrete responsibility, every concrete decision, striving to become responsible has to fold out this paradox, not by solving it but through de-paradoxification making the impossible look possible, that is referring to the general in a personal way hiding the reference. It is a game of invisibilisation of the logic of repetition; making invisible that the absolute repeat the general. Ethics (general responsibility), says Derrida, is a temptation that absolute responsibility has to resist:

> The ethical therefore ends up making us irresponsible. It is a temptation, a tendency, or a facility that would sometimes have to be refused in the name of responsibility that doesn't keep account or give account to man, to humans, to society, to one's fellows, or to one's self. Such a responsibility keeps it secret, it cannot and need not present itself.
>
> (Derrida 1992: 62)

Responsibilisation may lead to hyper-responsibility

Let's return to health dialogues, health partnerships and health games. They are about ascribing responsibility to the individual citizen, but how does this responsibility relate to the form of personal responsibility analysed by Kierkegaard and Derrida? We shall look at this issue in two ways. One is how health games actually violate the form of personal responsibility. The other is how a new form emerges, displacing personal responsibility with a kind of playful hyper-responsibility equivalent to heterophony.

If we ask how health dialogues, health partnerships and health games violate the form of personal responsibility, it is striking how they constantly produce ethical temptations for citizens. They offer citizens an easy way out of their personal responsibility by substituting personal responsibility with advice, dialogues and recipes. Health dialogues, health partnerships and health games only appeal to general responsibility and risk absolute and singular responsibility. Often they do not articulate expectations about specific responsible actions. Instead, citizens are tempted to break the secrecy that protects their absolute responsibility. When absolute responsibility announces itself in playful dialogues, it is no longer absolute; personal responsibility is no longer yours alone but ours. The health profession asks for more personal responsibility but does not really trust the citizens the capacity of singularity. They do not (like Kierkegaard's father) give personal responsibility time to mature or alternatively trust that personal responsibility is already present. They substitute it with public play, commitments and dialogues. And when citizens reject the temptations of ethics, health professionals do not regard citizens as responsible individuals but as self-powerless. Health professionals then try to tempt citizens in new ways, making responsibility easier to carry or just fun and playful. But the result is also a devaluation of expectations with regard to absolute responsibility. Citizens are no longer expected to have the capacity of being absolutely responsible. Like children, they are only in as long as it is funny and easy.

But there is another possible reading marking, that what is happening is a re-entry of the form creating hyper-responsibility (see Figure 4.3). General responsibility is doubled. General responsibility becomes itself a unity of a distinction. This distinction is drawn between a hypothetical, emergent and singular absolute responsibility, on the one hand, and a heterophonic surplus of general responsibilities, on the other. The unity of this distinction is general responsibility in the form of an ethics of potentiality and play.

Health dialogues, health partnerships and health games mark that it is no longer possible to articulate stable general expectations about responsibility. It has, of course, always been the case that there is a surplus of general responsibilities. But now general responsibility is produced in such a way that it reflects this surplus. Health professionals reflect that they cannot take responsibility for what health responsibility is. Health responsibility is too much, too many things and too indeterminate to be articulated as stable

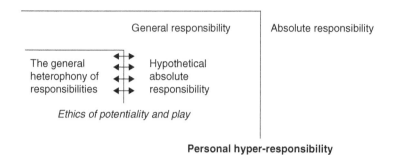

Figure 4.3 Hyper-responsibility.

rules or norms. By their very nature, health games indicate that general responsibility has become singular and bound to temporary processes. So, with health dialogues, partnerships and games, health professionals do not take responsibility for defining general responsibilities. Instead, they take responsibility for facilitating a process in which participants can investigate *potential* general responsibilities, and by marking this process 'dialogue', 'a promise about a later promise' or 'play', the temporary and singular of the general is underlined. So we get an ethics of potentiality that defines general responsibility as a heterophonic reservoir of possible responsibilities. It is also an ethics of play because it invites a playful oscillation between codes, investigating potential responsibilities.

What is then expected of absolute responsibility? Well, it is not simply expected to be a responsible decision and act. What is expected primarily is self-investigation of the possible relations between the absolute and the general, and, when the general has become emergent and singular (on the temporal dimension), the only possibility with regard to acting with absolute responsibility is to be playful and take part in the responsibility games and dialogues. In the past, health authorities acted as experts, formulating answers, rules and norms, expecting individuals to be absolutely responsible. Now authorities experience that their answers cannot be formulated in a sufficiently general way. On the other hand, they do not dare to leave the responsibility for health to individuals and their personal responsibility. Therefore, they mark the personal responsibility that used to be unmarked. They aim at regulating personal responsibility, marking it as a public responsibility to create personal responsibility. This means the personal responsibility is both marked as a public matter and at the same time has to be presumed personal. We get a re-entry of the distinction, forming on its inner side a second order responsibility, an ethic of potentiality, investigating relations between general and absolute. And, on the outer side of the distinction, a yet unmarked and incommunicable absolute responsibility.

As Figure 4.3 seeks to show, the form of hyper-responsibility is a new general responsibility defining responsibility as an investigation of potential responsibilities. So general responsibility goes second order and involves the responsibility for an open investigation of pontential responsibility. Ethics of potentiality and play is one of second order. This responsibility to investigate through dialogues, partnerships and games involves both an investigation of the heterophonic reservoir of possible responsibilities (what does responsibility look like in this code, in that code, etc.) and an investigation of potential absolute responsible ways to answer or not answer general responsibilities (the arrows). So the hypothetical absolute responsibilities in the form of potentiality become reflexive and second-order. And all the time, an unmarked side of hyper-responsibility is always implied as the non-hypothetical absolute responsibility.

Conclusion

We argue that the current call for responsibilisation of the citizen can be understood as a way to meet the challenge of heterophony. The health system tries both to address health responsibilities and to suspend the same responsibilities in order to leave room for other system perspectives as the health system realises that it depends on factors in the educational system, the economic system, the love system, etc. Responsibilisation of the individual is turned into a strange kind of steering medium with the purpose of balancing and linking various systemic perspectives. The individual is imagined a possible nexus of perspectives. A governing challenge occurs that can only be met by the individual taking a personal responsibility for taking all the possible duties into consideration and deciding which ones are the most important. However, the health system doesn't trust the individual to be thorough enough without guidance; personal responsibility seems to be too serious a matter to be left to the individual. But how should individuals be governed with a view to making them personally responsible?

A number of creative social technologies are designed to handle these paradoxical steering ambitions. Technologies are designed as a monological call for dialogue with patients about their approach to personal responsibility. Oscillating between unilateral monologue and mutual dialogues, the potentiality of responsibilisation in the different coding is investigated. On top of dialogues, partnerships are designed as a technology that can investigate the capacity of commitments in different codings. The basic machine in partnership is the constant oscillation between binding and non-binding obligations turning agreements second-order by only promising later promises. And, finally, health games are designed as a prescription for play functioning as a technology to bring in more imaginary capacity to the dialogues and partnerships. The games are a kind of potentiality accelerators.

What happens to personal responsibility in these paradoxical communications? In order to answer this question we read the analysis of personal responsibility by Søren Kierkegaard and Jacques Derrida in a systems-the-oretical way. We conceptualise personal responsibility by asking what the structure of expectation regarding personal responsibility is. What should you as an individual expect of yourself with a view to regarding yourself as personally responsible in a modern Western context? This way of posing the question has not been approached by systems theory before now. Systems theory has either discussed personal responsibility as something to be attrib-uted in the communication or personal responsibility has been observed as a question posed in moral communication where the communication takes the form of recognition/misrecognition. By focusing on the expect-ation structure we can point to the impossibility embedded in the form of personal responsibility, the form being that you have to meet both external duties, ethics, norms and follow your inner voice in order to be regarded as personally responsible. We can show how the call for heterophony and the ambition to make citizens personally responsible, for example for their own health, leads to a second-order personal responsibility where you have to reflect in public on the impossibility of meeting both external and internal duties. This, we argue, involves a displacement of the form of the category of personal responsibility. A playful form of second-order hyper-responsibility emerges as an answer to heterophony. This does not substitute the original form of personal responsibility but doubles it, creating a rather complex discursive game where absolute responsibility is both a hypothetic elem-ent in the ethic of potentiality and still an unmarked presumption of the whole game.

Notes

1 See http://www.legdigsund.dk.
2 See http://www.legdigsund.dk.
3 See http://www.legdigsund.dk.

References

Andersen, N. Å. (2004) 'The Contractualisation of the Citizen: On the Transformation of Obligation into Freedom', in *Social Systems*, 10 (2): 273–91.
——(2007) 'Creating the Client Who Can Create Himself and His Own Fate: The Tragedy of the Citizens' Contract', *Qualitative Sociology Review*, 3 (2): 119–43.
——(2008a) 'The World as Will and Adaptation: The Inter-Discursive Coupling of Citizens' Contracts', *Critical Discourse Studies*, 5 (1): 75–89.
——(2008b) *Partnerships: Machines of Possibilities*, Bristol: The Policy Press.
——(2009) *Power at Play: The Relationships Between Play, Work and Governance*, Basingstoke: Palgrave Macmillan.
——(2011) 'Who is Yum-Yum? A Cartoon State in the Making', *Ephimera, Theory and Politics in Organization*, 11 (4): 406–32.
Baecker, D. (1999) 'The Form Game', in D. Baecker (ed.), *Problems of Form*, Palo Alto, Calif.: Stanford University Press, pp. 99–107.

Bateson, G. (1955) 'The Message "This Is Play"', in B. Schaff (ed.), *Group Processes, Transactions of the Second Conference October 9, 10, 12, 1955*, Princeton, NJ: Josiah Macy J.R. Foundation, pp. 145–242.

——(2000) *Steps to an Ecology of Mind: Collected Essays in Anthropology, Psychiatry, Evolution, and Epistemology*, Chicago, Ill.: University of Chicago Press.

Danish Society for General Medicine (2001) *Den motiverende samtale: Klaringsrapport nr. 1*, Copenhagen.

Danish Committee for Health Education (2005) *The Hash Dialogue*, Copenhagen.

Danish Medicines and Health Authority (2007) *Socialt udsatte borgeres sundhed–barrierer, motivation og muligheder*, Copenhagen.

——(2002) *10 gode grunde til IKKE at forebygge!*, Copenhagen.

——(2010) *Sundhed i beskæftigelsesindsatsen*, Copenhagen.

Danish Medicines and Health Authority, Danish Ministry of Education, Danish National Council for Children, and Danish Committee for Health Education (2005) 'Børn, unge og alkohol. Information til forældre', Copenhagen.

Danish Veterinary and Food Administration, National Board of Health and School and Society (2007) *Sundhed på spil – dialog og samarbejde om klassens sundhed, et spil*, Copenhagen.

Derrida, J. (1988) *The Ear of the Other*, Lincoln, Nebr.: University of Nebraska Press.

——(1992) *The Gift of Death*, Chicago, Ill.: The University of Chicago Press.

——(2007) 'Des tours de Babel', in J. Derrida (ed.), *Psyche: Inventions of the Other*, vol. I. Palo Alto, Calif.: Stanford University Press, pp. 191–225.

Gadamer, H.-G. (1985) *Truth and Method*, New York: The Crossroad Publishing Company.

Højlund, H. and L. T. Larsen (2001) 'Det sunde fællesskab', *Distinktion: Scandinavian Journal of Social Theory*, 3 (3): 73–90.

Kierkegaard, S. (1946) *Either/or*, vol. II, London: Oxford University Press.

Knudsen, H. (2009) 'The Betwixt and Between Family Class', *Nordic Educational Review*, 29 (1): 149–62.

——(2010) *Har vi en aftale?*, Frederiksberg: Nyt fra Samfundsvidenskaberne.

——(2011) 'The Game of Hospitality', *Ephemera, Special Issue on Work, Play and Boredom*, 11 (4): 433–49.

Knudsen, H. and N. Å. Andersen (2014) 'Playful Hyper-responsibility: Toward a Dislocation of Parents' Responsibility?' *Journal of Education Policy*, 29 (1): 105–21.

Luhmann, N. (1987) 'The Morality of Risk and the Risk of Morality', *International Review of Sociology*, 3 (3): 87–101.

——(1990) *Political Theory in the Welfare State*, New York: Walter de Gruyter.

——(1993) 'The Code of Moral', *Cardozo Law Review*, 14 (4): 995–1009.

——(1995) *Social Systems*, Palo Alto, Calif.: Stanford University Press.

Michailakis, D. and W. Schirmer (2010) 'Agents of Their Health? How the Swedish Welfare State Introduces Expectations of Individual Responsibility', *Sociology of Health and Illness*, 32 (6): 930–47.

Ministry of Food, Agriculture and Fisheries (2008) www.legdigsund.dk.

Ministry of Health (1999) *Regeringens Folkesundhedsprogram, 1999–2008*, Copenhagen.

Monthoux, P. G. de and M. Statler (2008) 'Aesthetic Play As an Organizing Principle', in D. Barry and H. Hansen (eds.), *The Sage Handbook of New Approaches in Management and Organization*, London: Sage Publications, pp. 423–35.

Nullmeier, F. (2006) 'Personal Responsibility and Its Contradiction in Terms', *German Policy Studies*, 3 (3): 386–99.

Rasmussen, B. M. and H. Toft (2005) *Udviklingshæmmede og misbrug: metodeudvikling på tværs af sektorer*, CVU Sødnerjylland.

Rose, N. (1999) *Powers of Freedom: Reframing Political Thought*, Cambridge: Cambridge University Press.

Stichweh, R. (1997) 'Professions in Modern Society', *International Review of Sociology*, 7 (1): 95–102.

Part III

Organisational arrangements

5 Arranging medical and economic logics

Investigating the influence of economic controlling in an internal medicine department

Werner Vogd

Introduction

German hospitals are currently undergoing profound transition. The introduction in January 2003 of diagnosis-related groups (DRGs) led to a fundamental change in the settlement of performances. The main basis for financing was no longer the length of stay but a flat-rate charge for each type of case.

At the same time, and often in connection with the privatisation of hospitals, modern management techniques were introduced, with computer-based financial controlling, outsourcing and centralisation of key operational functions.

This means that the economic logic also becomes apparent for the medical personnel and thus becomes unavoidable in the daily processes. This does not imply that medicine was not previously an economic fact, namely in the sense that resources were to be mobilised for treatment and diagnosis (and also that these were always limited). The new feature in the present situation, however, is that the economic integration is not only experienced as a general limitation of resources but that the economic reflection now permeates through all areas of medical treatment and care. The economic and the medicinal logic can no longer simply be uncoupled under these circumstances, for example in the sense that the doctor was responsible primarily for the medicine and the hospital manager for the acquisition of the resources, with only loose ties due to the separation of personal responsibilities. Rather, the increased possibilities for financial controlling in medicine mean that economic considerations are taken into account in every specific case, in every diagnostic and therapeutic decision. Medicine and economics are therefore always simultaneously present under the given conditions. There are also possible legal consequences where a doctor can be shown to have breached medical codes, and in recent years there has been a considerable increase in the requirements for documentation (and therefore the traceability) of medical actions in addition to the increased economic documentation. The question is how the organisation hospital can reach some arrangement between the often incommensurable economic, medical and legal demands under such tightened reflective conditions.

These processes could not only change the context of physicians' actions but could also influence their decision-making processes, probably to a not-inconsiderable extent. In addition, tensions are to be expected between the traditional behaviour of physicians and the new organisational demands.

The consequences of these processes for the daily work of physicians was reconstructed on the basis of field observations and topic-centred interviews on a surgical and an internal medicine ward of two German urban hospitals in a qualitative longitudinal study.[1] In the period from January 2000 to January 2002, four field research visits were made to two urban hospitals and two university clinics (Vogd 2004b). In 2004, the urban hospitals were revisited.[2]

The empirical material was evaluated according to the documentary method of Ralf Bohnsack (2003b), taking into account frames and framing processes.[3] The processes of change and their interactive dynamics were reconstructed in a three-level comparative analysis. After an initial pre-post comparison, the second level involves the comparison of observations or reconstructions from various medical disciplines and cultures. The third level then concentrates on the relationship of observed actions and the comments made by the medical actors. By contrasting in this way, it was possible to develop the tensions between the routines of the doctors and the new organisational requirements in respect to the different institutional logics and to analyse the importance of these dissonances for the shaping of the transformation processes (cf. Vogd 2006).[4]

In the following presentation of the partial results of these studies, the focus is on the implicit knowledge involved in the medical actions and, second, on an organisation-sociology perspective which is not restricted to negotiation processes and micro-political games but which also takes into account the specialities of a functionally differentiated society in general and its medicine in particular. This raises empirically the question how the different logics of the function systems (especially medicine, economy, law) could be set into a workable arrangement. Since the relationship between a praxeological and a system-theoretical perspective is not immediately apparent, some organisation-sociological and methodological remarks follow on the conceptual and meta-theoretical framework of the project. This is followed by a consideration of the changing economic conditions for hospitals and then the changing organisation of the work of physicians. In the section on professional ethos, the unfolding actions of doctors in a medically complex case are considered in their organisational context. The concluding discussion then compares and contrasts the empirical inferences and sociological theories.

Under the given conditions, it is increasingly necessary to make use of networks and the relationship forms expressed in them in order to process the paradoxes and contradictions that arise due to the presence of differing logics.

Organisational sociology and methodology

The reconstruction of processes in organisations such as hospitals is not straightforward. It is not sufficient to view what happens in terms of the 'negotiated order' (Strauss *et al.* 1963) or the expert power (Freidson 1970). In spite of the insights offered by the interactionist perspective, it does not take into account all the structural constraints and the degrees of freedom of organisations.

According to conventional organisation theory, organisations as 'corporative actors' are aimed at fulfilling a certain purpose. The problem is then how the individual actors can be brought to coordinate their efforts effectively, although as members of the organisation they each pursue their own goals, which do not necessarily coincide with the purpose of the organisation. Also, organisations like hospitals don't show only one rationality but are, as an institutional order, committed to different logics. Freidson, for example, points out that medical institutions are at once framed by *bureaucratism*, *economism* and *professionalism* (cf. Freidson 2001).

In system theory, an organisation is a unit that reproduces itself simply in terms of its own system rationality, on the basis of its own operations. Furthermore, organisations are social units that observe themselves and can determine their own functional relationships, in other words their remit, by means of internal decisions (cf. Luhmann 2000b).

Organisations will usually link themselves to a social functional system, for example, the hospital to the medical system. However, the systemic reproductive framework of an organisation should not be viewed as identical with the functional setting in question.

From the perspective of system theory, it is not likely that the performances offered by the organisations of the medical system are optimally adapted to its functions. Rather, it is to be expected that there are tensions within the organisations between purposive and system rationality. What may appear to be purposive-rational is not necessarily rational in terms of its systemic implementation. Viewed empirically, organisations in this sense represent a 'meeting place' of the functional systems (Luhmann 2000a: 398), with an organisation relating to the legal, economic, medical and other semantics each in its own way.

From the perspective of system theory, there is a difference between organisation systems and interaction systems. Physicians may distance themselves in their interactions from the goals of their organisation, for example by standing up for their medical remit in informal communications against the decisions of the hospital management or by entering into a complicit alliance with the patients to simulate certain diagnoses and therapies in order to ensure the finances for the measures considered necessary.

As shown by our previous investigation of the decision behaviour of physicians (Vogd 2004b), a key characteristic of the communication of doctors in hospitals is the search for a balance between medical, organisational and economic contextures. As already shown by Parsons (1951), the treatment of patients can only be established as a sustainable social system if the patient can expect, or in the sense of Luhmann can trust, that the illness is the focus of concern, and not money or the pursuit of intimate relationships.[5] Conversely, the doctor will only feel able to carry out brutal and shameless diagnostic and therapeutic procedures if it can be assumed that the patients are concerned with the therapy and not with law or a non-hierarchical discourse. For medical treatment, both sides must assume that medicine forms the 'primary framework' (Goffman) and is to be understood as the situation definition which allows that actual to appear (Goffman 1986: 31 ff.). With Luhmann, it is possible to abstract Goffman's framework concept from the point of view of the individual actor to a socio-theoretical setting. A framework now corresponds to a specific societal contexture that follows a coherent logic in which specific classes of communicative connections are possible. The point of Luhmann's social analysis is that the modern society is poly-contextual, with different, overlapping functional logics for the economy, the legal system, science and medicine, and with organisation and interaction systems that are conditioned by their own history.[6]

Whereas in pre-modern medicine the treatment and the consequence of no treatment were discussed in face-to-face interaction, for example, between monarch and personal physician, or peasant and itinerant healer, the modern doctor–patient relationship is also embedded in legal, economic, political and scientific contexts, each with causalities that are independent of this relationship. The doctor and patient cannot affect whether the cost of a proposed therapy will be met by the health-insurance company or whether passive euthanasia is legal. At this point, organisations once again play a role. Although structurally above interaction, the hospital as an organisation is neither subsumed by its medical purpose nor by economic rationality or the administrative implementation of policies or legal requirements. The performance of organisations is to gain degrees of freedom in the internal-external difference in order to bring together the different societal expectation structures. The hospital is often only able to do justice to the economic logic by circumventing this, for example, by submitting accounts with diagnoses in an 'as if' mode, in order to carry out medical measures which are viewed as necessary but which would not be payable. The hospital is able to provide terminally ill patients with palliative care while doing justice to the administrative and medical logic with (medically senseless) diagnosis and therapy (cf. Vogd 2002). Legal requirements are met by presenting written documentation of the case history that obscures all the smaller infringements which are demanded by 'practical reason' (Bourdieu) under time pressure.

At a more general level, there are links to investigations in the field of so-called new institutionalism. It is also possible to show how organisations gain additional *degrees of freedom* by functionally decoupling the sectors of the organisation (cf. DiMaggio and Powell 1991), so that, for example, the quality assurance only evaluates the documentation but looks less closely at the practice (Power 1997; for the medical system in particular see Scott *et al.* 2000).

Methods

The documentary method conceived by Ralf Bohnsack (2003a) and further developed by Vogd (2004b, 2011) as a method for organisation research provides an instrument to reconstruct the above-mentioned processes in their modus operandi, as well as the associated framing processes.[7] The methodology is in accordance with Luhmann's time relationship inasmuch as the propositional content of a statement is only determined *post hoc* by means of the framing chosen in the communicative connections.

The demanding task of carrying out reconstructive organisation research not only from the perspective of interaction theory but also of social theory can now be tackled by an empirical approach to the question of the relevant structures. Bohnsack speaks of 'meaningful genesis' and the socio-genesis of these structures.

These processes can only be reconstructed by extensive comparative analysis in which the *tertium comparationis* is systematically displaced, which is treated in each case as dependent or independent variable and changed with regard to possible socio-genetic conditional factors.

In this way, it is finally possible to obtain a multidimensional typology with which the investigated phenomena can be described as an overlapping of various orientations (cf. Bohnsack 2001). Only such an approach does justice to the complexity of organisations in which not only do the contextures of societal function systems meet but in which there are also multiple internal differentiations in hierarchies, vocational groups, milieus and various spheres of communication.

In particular, the view of the development of the medical departments over time clearly shows how the 'organisation hospital' can preserve its autonomy from its societal surroundings (not only policy-makers but also the patients and their relatives), which orientations are invariant and will be maintained even in the event of considerable staff cuts and changing modes of accounting, and new phenomena which are to be expected (such as shifts in the network's complexity).

In the following, the partial results of the longitudinal study are presented. The methodology of this study has already been presented variously elsewhere and is not repeated here. In order to allow depth of description, I limit myself here to the restudy of the department of internal medicine.

Changing economic framework

During the first period of investigation in 2001, the clinics in question were still in public-sector ownership, but shortly afterwards they were taken over by private holding companies. This led to reorganisation, in which medical departments were merged and management functions centralised. Modern office technology was introduced so that doctors could use monitors, keyboards and databases to access patient data, correspondence, laboratory values, etc.

In both departments, there were cutbacks of 25–30 per cent in the numbers of physicians. As a consequence of changes to the definitions of forms of duty, the reorganisation of night shifts and cuts in the special Christmas and holiday payments, the doctors in both hospitals suffered salary cuts of 20–25 per cent in comparison with 2001.

A significant structural change was the revision of the method of cost calculations. Hospital charges are no longer based on the length of the hospital stay but rather on the flat-rate system of the DRGs. The DRG system was developed in the 1970s in the USA by Robert Fetter and was introduced there in the 1980s with the political goal of reducing the length of patient stays in American hospitals.

The preconditions for the relevant coding of a patient within the DRG system is, first, the coding of a main diagnosis and related diagnoses in the ICD (International Classification of Diseases) code and the procedures carried out on the patients which can be represented in the ICPM (International Classification of Procedures in Medicine) code. On the basis of the diagnoses and procedures as well as the age, sex, length of stay and type of dismissal (e.g., normal, transferred, deceased), a DRG is then determined by means of a computer algorithm. For each DRG, a relative weighting is calculated with which the revenues from various DRGs can be compared. It must be emphasised that the DRGs are primarily an economic classification rather than a medical one, because in the treatment process a series of procedures may prove to be important which cannot be reflected in the coding system. For most DRGs, an upper and lower limit is set for the length of stay in the hospital. Money is withheld if a stay is too short in order to avoid rewarding 'red' dismissals. Only if the length of stay significantly exceeds the average, an extra payment is made to cover complications. Periods are also defined within which a repeated admission to a hospital is not paid for. This is intended to prevent hospitals from dividing up a treatment process into a series of steps which can be charged to a number of different DRGs. The individual revenues for a DRG are reduced if a patient is treated by two or more hospitals. The need for 'cost equality' (a by-no-means-trivial consideration both economically and in terms of practical organisational considerations) leads to constant changes to the coding regulations.

The intention is that the DRG system in its current form should reward treatments with short stays that do not require any further admissions. The computerised DRG coding also opens up various possibilities for medical data-processing. For any specific case, each doctor can see on the computer if the case promises a profit with respect to the length of stay or threatens a loss. Furthermore, in external and internal hospital surveys, individual departments, wards, teams or even individual physicians can be compared and subjected to benchmark testing.

The DRG system makes a difference in the hospital because it makes the economic contexture for the doctors visible. It forces the daily work processes immediate to align with economic constrain.

Organisation of the work of physicians

At first sight, there seem to have been no major changes to the structure and organisation of the internal medicine department in 2004 compared with the first observation period. Resident physicians continue to supervise the wards. The functional diagnostics and registration draw on their own teams of co-workers. The numbers of nursing staff on the ward have remained constant. However, whereas in 2001 there were 3.75 physicians for thirty-six patients in the ward under observation, three years later, only 2.25 doctors are allocated for the same number of beds. At the same time, the average stay of a patient has shortened over this period from eleven to seven days, intensifying the workload for the doctors. The medical personnel can only cope with the personnel cuts and the higher turnover of patients by maintaining a constantly high work rate.

In effect, two doctors now share responsibility for a ward with thirty-six beds. As a consequence of holidays, days off and gaps caused by night duty, there are days when only one of the physicians is on duty, and sometimes neither of them is present. This can mean that a colleague from the neighbouring ward or the functional department has to stand in.

On the wards, a distinction is made between problem cases and routine cases. In contrast with the past, the latter are now only superficially examined. Whereas in 2001 every patient on the ward was examined again thoroughly by the resident physician, who could thus become personally acquainted with the patient and the case, this is only possible as an exception under current conditions. The doctors now rely on the diagnosis given by the colleague on the admission ward. There are now much fewer group visits, and the information handed over to the physician starting the next shift is, as a rule, solely in the written form. However, the increased reliance on the written form does not correlate with improved patient documentation, because under the burden of routine work the ward doctors have less time to make detailed and orderly entries on the patient charts. Since gaps have to be left at all levels, the doctors must make practical decisions about medical priorities and where they feel it is justifiable to risk omissions.

A patient will usually be without a physician's supervision during the absence from the ward of the colleague who admitted them. Only in emergencies will the stand-in physician work through the unfamiliar documentation. In phases when the duty roster means that there are frequent changes of personnel, it is necessary to find interim solutions in order to ensure that the gaps in the medical care are not unacceptably large. Because often only one ward doctor is present for the ward round of the chief physician and senior physicians, they often meet patients who are unknown to the ward doctor.

Since the senior physicians also have less time to accompany the chief physician around the wards, the character and function of the chief physician's rounds change. They no longer appear before the patient as a decision-making team discussing treatment options. The rounds now function rather as a control in which the chief physicians can take decisions concerning the particularly problematic cases. The increased workload and the lower staffing ratios mean that the ward physicians are responsible for taking more decisions. The shorter treatment cycles mean that it is no longer possible for every decision to be confirmed by the team.

The time allocated for routine procedures is often so short that the responsible physician can no longer thoroughly inspect the patient, for example, before and after a cardiac catheterisation. It was observed on various occasions that a patient was discharged after a cardiological intervention without having been seen even once by the responsible ward doctor signing the discharge.

The new conditions involve a division of labour which means that the physician can only establish a personal clientele relationship by way of an exception. The old habitus of the internal physician as the philosopher and interpreter of disease does reoccur, in particular in complex cases, but in the majority of routine cases decisions are made on the basis of the file and standard diagnostic procedures. Expertise is only deployed when cases are problematic and call for more intensive communications and reflection (see the following section).

In contrast to the past, the medical logic is now clearly dissociated from the logic of settlement. Since the DRG system does not reward the clarification of various syndromes, a discrepancy arises between the orientation of internal medicine to clarify the various differential diagnoses and the requirement to concentrate on the main diagnosis of the DRG.

This leads to a class of situations in which, for example, the internal physician sees the priority as the search for a tumour as a result of the patient's anaemia but in which it would be better to enter a DRG code for a cardiac infarct in the sense of covering costs. The organisational considerations make it necessary for the physicians to adopt the best paid medically plausible coding. In particular, in complicated cases it is not only necessary to encode the secondary diagnoses and the various procedures involved, which itself can be extremely time-consuming, but the physicians must also decide which main diagnosis promises the best payment. In parallel, a letter of discharge has to be carefully formulated in order to avoid giving the impression of manipulation to increase profits. In the case of 'multi-morbid' patients, it can take thirty to forty minutes until the coding is finished and the doctor's letter has been written (cf. also Vogd 2006: 77 ff.).

Considering the problems of complex cases, it will now be considered how the new economic parameters have changed the medical orientation of physicians.

Maintaining professional ethos

Following on from previous investigations (cf. Vogd 2004b: 289 ff.), complex cases are those involving medically demanding treatment processes. As a rule, extensive, and often expensive, diagnostic procedures are necessary in order to eliminate other possibilities and finally to arrive at a medically based decision. Such cases often lead to a cascade of subsequent organisational or administrative problems and require further decisions. The key question for physicians is whether to deploy the full range of state-of-the-art medical techniques or to restrict themselves to a narrow range of procedures at the risk of discharging the patient without complete diagnostic clarification. These cases seem to be particularly relevant for the consideration here of the essence and ethos of good medical practice. Consideration of the problems of complex cases can show which aspects of the doctors' actions and orientations are negotiable and which are integral parts of medical practice. Methodologically, treatment processes from the two observation periods are compared and contrasted. In one case, a patient who had been part of the study in 2001 was coincidentally also admitted to the internal medicine ward three years later during the second observation period ('Herr Spondel'). It should not be assumed that this necessarily provides grounds for a thematic comparison, but in this case it became apparent after only a few observation sessions that the second treatment process also constituted a 'complex case', which justified the potentially interesting comparison.

The reconstruction of the events from 2001 has already been published (Vogd 2004a, 2004b, 2011), so the presentation here begins with a short reconstruction of the cases from 2004.[8] All names have been changed to protect those involved.

Herr Spondel, seventy-six years old, is transferred to the hospital on a Monday evening by Dr Reinhardt, a nephrologist with a dialysis surgery close to the clinic. The doctor, who is very familiar with the procedures in the hospital, arranges for the patient to be given a nuclear medical investigation, without a resident physician being consulted. Before the ward doctor, Dr Kardel, arrives at work the next morning, the patient has already been called up for the investigation. The duty doctor says to the observer that this represents a catastrophe, because the procedure is very complicated and expensive. In addition, she had not seen either the patient or his file:

Tuesday, 11 August, 8.40 a.m. (in the corridor)
DR KARDEL (TO THE OBSERVER): This morning we already have the 'Ultimate-MCA' (maximum credible accident) … Herr Spondel… comes here to the dialysis surgery of … [Dr] Rheinhardt, he transferred the patient to this ward … and this morning he was taken for a long-term scintigraphy… that is very complicated and expensive investigation… I was supposed to sign for it, although I have seen neither the patient nor the file … of course

I didn't [sign] ... now he is downstairs receiving the investigation ... I don't know who will sign the form for it now ...

OBSERVER: What sort of investigation is that?

DR KARDEL: You need it to localise sources of inflammation ... radioactively tagged leukocytes enrich at a source of inflammation ... his own leukocytes are removed first ... they have to be his own ...

Dr Kardel begins with a superlative of the term 'maximum credible accident' from technology assessments, which in German is widely used in a metaphorical sense. But although the lay person might expect this to refer to an irreversible medical error, it is used about an expensive investigation which was instigated by an external physician, sidestepping the regular decision-making structures of the organisation. The physician has no choice but to legitimise the investigation *post hoc* by signing the form. The real catastrophe here is, first, that the autonomy of the organisation, which in Luhmann's terms reproduces itself by its own internal decisions, has been undermined through informal channels. Second, at the personal level, she will sign as ward physician for an expensive procedure which may not have been necessary.

Dr Kardel faces a dilemma. If she signs for the investigation retrospectively, she will assume responsibility for it. If she refuses to sign, she discloses the scandal that the investigation was not the result of legitimate decisions. But this will be disloyal to the people who made the procedure possible through their informal assistance. This could be a problem, since she may in future depend on the benevolence of the radiology department, the nurses and the duty staff to achieve an informal solution for some other problem.

When these two approaches are considered together, it becomes apparent that something has happened here which really can be referred to as an 'accident'. The delicate arrangement between formal and informal communication, with official lines of decision-making and informal personal interactions on the basis of trust seem here to have broken down. In this sense the doctor does not measure the event in terms of moral categories but frames it as a technical accident.

At this stage, we do not know about the medical background of the unfolding drama, but we can intuit that this example may touch the heart of the action and decision dynamics of the modern hospital. On the one hand, there is the economic burden on the department of a cost-intensive radiological investigation. On the other hand, there are likely to be medical considerations, because otherwise why should Dr Rheinhardt, the external nephrologist, undertake this ingression into the centre of an organisation?

A little later, the doctor studies the file of the new patient. She reads out some of the details. A listening colleague comments that he had no idea that the expensive investigation would go through with no way of stopping it. The doctor continues to study the file, formulates some diagnostic ideas and orders some additional laboratory investigations. She then visits the patient.

Herr Spondel is asked about his complaints and examined. She explains to the patient that some more investigations will follow and that they do not know how long he will have to stay.

In the corridor, Dr Kardel comments that this is a 'hard nut' to 'crack'. She looks in the file again and reads out loud. She then notices that, a few years previously, the patient had suffered inflammation of the vertebral body and that under these circumstances the leukocyte scintigraphy made sense. Her colleague, who happened to be standing in front of the ward room, added that bone scintigraphy might have been a better diagnostic option:

In the corridor

DR KARDEL: Well, that will be a hard nut to crack … [looks at the 'Red List' of approved drugs for some of the medication prescribed by the colleague] … that is the analgesic [names the product]

DR ELWERT: That is addictive …

DR KARDEL: It says as required … but I can't withdraw it just like that … [continues to look at the file in front of the ward room] … had spondylodiscitis … now pain again in that region … I am going to take a CT [computer tomography] …

DR ELWERT: … Yes, definitely …when did he have it?

DR KARDEL: [looks in the file] 01 …the leukocyte scintigraphy does makes sense, if he now has pain there …

DR ELWERT: Perhaps bone scintigraphy would be even better … [further discussion of both doctors about the patient]

Step by step, the doctor takes on the patient. As is usual in medical work, the physician's actions and decisions are prestructured by the medical file (cf. Berg 1996). Usually, a second step will then involve asking the patient personally about his complaints, with a short examination. While routine cases then are on track for a clear diagnosis and therapy, the metaphor of a 'tough nut' indicates that the patient is a complicated case, which, according to the chief physician, 'all doctors on the ward must be informed about'. The patient is now framed as a 'complex case', and in this case the second ward doctor participates in the discourse 'organically' and without being called on explicitly to do so. Within this special medical framing, the externally instigated radiological examination appears in a different light, namely as an appropriate way to 'crack the nut'. Further procedures are now also justified, such as CT.

As in the case three years earlier, the doctors also appear to be willing, under the new conditions, to go to greater lengths in this complicated case, and the medical criteria take priority over organisational and economic considerations.

The doctor enters on the top sheet of the medical file the known diagnoses and the diagnostic procedures. The probable duration of stay is given as fourteen days.

The top sheet now includes:

- X-ray, prone: large pleural effusion
- Sonography → aerobilia, splenomegaly
- CT-Lumbar spine/sacrum

Yellow sheet:

- Transfer diagnosis: R 63.4 Abnormal loss of weight
- Admission diagnosis: One-sided pleural effusion

Further diagnoses:

- Abnormal loss of weight
- Infection (previous)
- Terminal renal insufficiency
- Congestive cardiac insufficiency
- Probable duration of stay: fourteen days

It is evident to even the lay observer that the patient is suffering from so-called multimorbidity. In contrast to three years previously, the documentation includes the planned length of stay and the DRG coding for the admission diagnosis.

There are noticeable discrepancies between the transfer diagnosis of 'abnormal weight loss', the admission diagnosis 'one-sided pleural effusion' and the intended radiological clarification of the inflammation in the lower back. These all have different implications, using differing intra- and extra-organisational contextures. The diagnosis of 'abnormal loss of weight' can be said to represent the entrance ticket to the hospital, because it immediately suggests a possible cancer disease that requires admission for stationary clarification. The pleural effusion corresponds to the patient's obvious symptom. The clarification of the suspicion of a spondylodiscitis appears rather as a concealed objective, as the possible core of the hard nut, but it can only be carried out with considerable effort and should therefore not be mentioned to the medical controllers, because from the point of view of the organisation of the hospital, which is specialised in treating acute diseases, such chronic processes are not to be clarified further. The interaction of the various diagnoses no longer seems coincidental but are rather an intelligent communicative adaptation to the different systemic contextures. As in the procedures three years previously, the doctors gain autonomy with respect to the administrative constraints by modulating the framework in which a case appears.

Over lunch, a colleague reports about another department which has run up a deficit of €300,000. The senior physician replies that with Herr Spondel they have also got such a case in their ward. The problem is that the easy cases, which receive a simple routine treatment, were dealt with on an out-patient basis, whereas the cost-intensive difficult patients landed on the wards.

At this point it is clear that the doctors are aware of the economic dilemmas they face with complex cases. However, as will be seen later, the physicians' reflections about the systemic contextures do not lead to them dispensing with what is felt to be diagnostically or therapeutically necessary. In the afternoon, the ward doctor phones the radiological department to arrange a CT and is told that she will have to wait at least six days. The doctor replies that it might be better to order a magnetic resonance tomography (MRT) because that would probably be available much more quickly.

Under the new conditions of the DRG-coded flat-rate system, a treatment process now seems to be a race against time. Whereas three years earlier a longer hospital stay had been economically desirable, provided that a plausible explanation could be given to the health insurer, the prime concern is now to release the patients again as quickly as possible, even in complex cases. The control parameter 'length of stay' led to the doctor considering whether to resort to the more expensive MRT investigation. The alternatives formulated here are significant. If the administration specifies the length of stay as a parameter for financial controlling, but on the other hand the capacities for routine diagnostics are limited, this does not mean at all that the doctors feel able to do without the corresponding 'medicine'. As can be seen from the observations of the surgical department (Vogd 2006), or from the conditions in America, the reduction of the durations of stays does not necessarily lead to increased economic rationality in the treatment processes. Whereas internal medicine often followed the principle of 'watch and wait', assuming that under careful clinical observation the solution would often present itself, time has become a limiting resource under the new conditions. This can mean that extensive, invasive and, in some cases, cost-intensive procedures are more attractive for the internal physician.

Over lunch, the doctor once again expresses amazement that Dr Rheinhardt could order a leukocyte scintigraphy externally and that the physician on duty had not even seen the patient beforehand. Dr Elwert remarks that as a physician on duty there is no longer enough time to bother with such things.

The colleague is arguing in terms of a time economy for the physician's attention. In view of the tighter rationing of the physicians' capacity, it is necessary to set priorities. It is not worth the time needed to work through the case history, because the next day the responsible ward physician will study the case more intensively anyway. From the point of view of the actors this is by no means irresponsible but an appropriate setting of priorities. A look at the referral diagnosis on the form from the admissions department shows that it is all right to wait until the next day. In an organisation with a highly developed division of labour, the judgement of the doctor in the admissions must be trusted. And one has to rely on the nurses to report any acute developments requiring the doctor to intervene.

In the afternoon, Dr Kardel informs the senior physician about the case. She mentions that Dr Rheinhardt had called for the leukocyte scintigraphy and that the patient had already been given up by another hospital. The senior physician replies that the case should be taken seriously and mentions that the patient has already 'messed up' the ward statistics once before. With the assessment by the senior physician, a coherent action framework has now been established. The medical orientation now forms the primary framework over and above other factors including economic considerations. The question of whether they want to give the patient a chance for the future and make the corresponding efforts means that the treatment process appears as one which involves a matter of life and death.

On the following Monday, the results of the leukocyte scintigraphy are available, and a written report on the X-ray examination of the pleural effusions. Dr Kardel phones to ask the X-ray department if they can take a sample of the pleural effusion of Herr Spondel during the pending CT. She explains to the observer that she has herself tried to take a sample during the sonography investigation, but this was not successful. Then the doctor talks to her colleague about the medication formulated in the doctor's referral letter. She notes that a mistake might have worked its way in regarding the doses and then been repeated in the various documents:

10.21 a.m. (in front of the ward room)
DR KARDEL (TO DR ELWERT): … are the dialysis medications still included?
    … now the erythropoietin … he receives a very high dose [gives a
    number] … in the letter from Rheinhardt there must be a text module
    error … because the mistake is repeated in the letter …

A doctor's work is based to large extent on the patient file with the documents recording past findings. It is remarkable in this case that the doctor is able to reflect on the contents of the file. The information cannot simply be taken at face value but must be examined for plausibility and consistency. The more technology involved in the process, the higher the potential for reflection must be.[9] With the term 'text module error', the doctor points to a new class of error for medicine which is caused by the computerisation of administrative tasks. Such artefacts will increase with the DRG system, not least because it dissociates medical and economic logic.

During the morning rounds, the patient mentions that he finds it difficult to breathe. The doctor listens to the breathing and then offers the patient another painkiller. In the corridor, she says to the observer that she has spoken with the senior physician on Friday about how much diagnostics one should carry out in this case. Since the patient has already had a carcinoma of the colon, one could look further in this direction. But it seems questionable whether another colonoscopy should be carried out because the patient is no longer 'in good shape'. The doctors here are faced with an elderly man who they do not wish to subject to the full array of diagnostic possibilities.

Here too there is a reflexive element. The diagnostic (and therapeutic) procedures no longer seem to be unconditionally good but have their own side effects. There are, therefore, two alternative pathways for medical treatment. Everything conceivable can be clarified in the sense of curative medicine, or a palliative approach can be adopted with the aim of relieving the symptoms somewhat. In both cases, however, the medical framing remains in the forefront. One is active in the interests of the patient. This is presumably why the doctor is willing to offer the patient something to relieve the pain.

While the chief physician is going around the ward the next day, the doctor presents Herr Spondel as an 'interesting case'.

Tuesday, 17 August, chief physician visits the ward

DR KARDEL: ... now an interesting case ... Herr Spondel... thick file ... dialysis patient ...

CHIEF PHYSICIAN: ... do we know him already?

DR KARDEL: ... switched from (Ward) 33 to 34 ... Pleural effusion ...attempt made to puncture ... now a CT ... again an attempt to puncture there ... they say it is not possible yet ... no fluid ... could now also be a mass ... a spondylodiscitis three years ago... but nothing to be seen now in the leukocyte scintigraphy ...

CHIEF PHYSICIAN: Now look at the 'Clinic' ...

DR KARDEL: Has pains in the lower back region ...

CHIEF PHYSICIAN: One should look at the CT now ... could be scarring perhaps ... the CRP [C-reactive protein, rises in response to inflammation] elevation can now also be non-specific ... could also be an infection now ... tuberculosis ... we should test ... a tuberculin sample ... and only if it is very quickly positive ... don't make things complicated all the time now, but think complexly ... in particular with infectious diseases ... they are coming back ...

In contrast to the facts produced by diagnostic procedures, the chief physician first draws attention to the so-called 'Clinic', meaning the symptom-related comments by the patient about how he feels. In the discussion of cases in internal medicine, it is often possible to observe the polarisation between 'clinical symptoms' and 'medical-diagnostic symptoms'. In particular in chronic cases, where there are often a variety of different diagnostic findings, it is possible in this way to reach a rapid decision. The inference can then be: 'If the patient is feeling all right despite unfavourable values and findings, then there is no reason to be precipitate with starting further activities.' From a functional perspective, the recourse to the 'Clinic' can also make it possible to cope with the complexity created in part by contradictory medical artefacts and findings. Since the survey of clinical symptoms, such as pains, represents a key element of the tradition of internal medicine, one remains here within the medical framework, in contrast to the recourse to the will of the patient (Vogd 2004b: 378 ff.).

The final remark of the chief physician is particularly noteworthy ('don't make things complicated all the time now but think complexly'). This expresses a core element of the philosophy of internal medicine. The main point is not so much actionism but rather a high degree of reflection about the work which has been done. A good doctor has an eye for both the potentialities and also the contingencies. However, which conclusions are to be drawn from this is another matter and can only be specified in the light of the conditions of the case at hand.

In his sense, the chief physician attempts to apply an holistic approach. A good doctor should have an overall view of medicine and, in case of doubt, should think beyond the well-trodden paths of the previous case history, for example considering a rare infectious disease. The recourse to the 'Clinic' can then be understood in another way. The orientation of the chief physician shows parallels to the first observation period, in which there were also sequences in the case of Herr Spondel when the chief physician tried to reduce the excessive complexity created by the ward physician. On the other hand, the approach of the chief physician indicates a potential solution to the economic-organisational dilemma in the treatment of complex cases. The trick is to keep the complexity in mind but then to take practical short cuts. There are signs of a shift in the orientation from the statements the chief physician made when doing the rounds in 2001.[10] The new internal physician would continue to think complexly but would no longer be able, as in the past, to clarify things in the full complexity.

In the afternoon, the ward physician phones Dr Rheinhardt, who referred the patient. She outlines the current considerations about the differential diagnosis and the planned further diagnostic procedures. The doctors also confer about how much the patient should be subjected to in terms of the further search for tumours.

The communication here about the reflection of the ongoing treatment extends beyond the organisational boundaries of the hospital. This is rather untypical of the first phase of observation and would normally form part of the follow-up after treatment. In this case, the referring doctor is involved in the internal discourse on the differential diagnosis as an important representative of the treatment network (see Freidson 1975). This shows the serious nature of the discourse about the patient. At a more fundamental level, this may also indicate a change in the organisation of the treatment process, towards a transorganisational treatment network.

After the phone call, Dr Kardel tells the observer that in the case of Herr Spondel she will also search for tumour markers. One should not really do that in such cases. But if there was a positive result then she would have a further reason to carry out a detailed intestinal examination. Tumour markers are substances produced by the body in response to cancer growth or by the cancer tissue itself. The problem is that the markers are often not specific enough, with too many false-positive results. If a number of markers are considered at the same time, then it is likely that a tumour would be indicated even in a healthy patient. The use of this diagnostic method is therefore also a performative act, because a positive result gives grounds to continue the search for a tumour (including invasive methods). In view of the psycho-social situation of the patient, an old man, certain diagnoses would have no therapeutic consequences. Nevertheless the trusted biomedical paradigm of maximum medicine implicitly calls for everything to be clarified without compromise. In its totality, this orientation may contradict both the economic-administrative primacy of the efficient use of resources (and also seem dubious from the perspective of the patient), but it seems that in particular in the complex cases, the 'medical gaze' (Foucault 2003) comes to itself.

In the following days, further investigations are conducted, but these do not lead to any definite results. On Thursday, the first results are received for the computer-supported puncture of the pleural effusion. The pathological finding describes a tumour process of undetermined origin. Additional tissue marking would make it possible to specify the diagnosis.

In the afternoon, the senior physician tells the doctor that there is now a definite finding. The patient has a mesenchymoma (a tissue carcinoma). However, this diagnosis has no therapeutic consequences. Rather, adequate pain control is called for. The ward physician then comments that the patient can be released at the start of the next week.

During the morning rounds the next day, the doctor asks the patient how he is feeling. Herr Spondel says that he has flickering in his eyes. The doctor suggests that he visit an ophthalmologist. She also explains that they have now identified 'malignant' cells but that in his condition they could not subject him to an operation. She explains that they now know where the symptoms are coming from. Finally, she asks the patient what care he has at home. Herr Spondel answers that his partner will care for him. The doctor enquires when he wants to be released and says that they could try to do what suited him. The patient suggests leaving after the weekend. He also describes the problems he has breathing. The doctor replies that this is because of the pleural effusion and they might also be able to give oxygen now. But first some tests will have to be carried out.

The situation is explained in an unspectacular way and with a gradual transition to palliative care, in which the priority emphasis is now on alleviating the symptoms. Surgery is now finally out of the question as a curative treatment option, but the doctor signals willingness to continue to act in the interests of the patient, who is allowed some autonomy about the time of dismissal – against the economic rationalities. He is also told that he can come back into hospital if need be. A little later, the doctor signs the form for the final X-ray investigation. The patient is finally released after a stay of twenty-one days in the hospital.

Discussion

Our investigations show that a hospital ward as a medical organisation is not subsumed in a commercial or macro-economic rationality, even under more stringent economic conditions and constraints on time and personnel. Rather, the medical orientation comes into its own and finds its highest expression in particular in the complicated cases. Correspondingly, when resources are restricted, the doctors distinguish between routine cases and difficult cases. For the former, it is medically justifiable to make omissions, whereas the organ systems of the latter receive the close attention. The same applies to the surgical department which was investigated. The comparative analyses show that this orientation is largely independent of the person who is ill. In other words, it will not depend on empathy or familiarity, nor on the special characteristics of a medical discipline or department. An unlikeable alcoholic will, as a rule, receive an equally high level of medical attention in the event of a suspected brain tumour (see Vogd 2006: 181 ff.).[11] The apparent homologies between the two processes are therefore not based on the recollection of the specific case and wish to give this person particularly good treatment but can be attributed to a generalisable medical orientation that manifests itself in complex cases by supporting the supposed interests of the patient against the economic interests of the organisation.

The patient is given a passive role in 2004 as in 2001. For example, whether Herr Spondel, as a multi-morbid patient, would want maximum medical treatment or would personally prefer to forgo invasive investigations is a question which is not asked within the constraints of modern medical treatment. Breaking out of these role expectations would require an exceptional display of will from a seriously ill individual, and within the treatment system it would usually be regarded as a disturbance (cf. Vogd 2004b: 365 ff.).

Against political correctness, it is easiest to sacrifice the attempts to democratise medical practice such as the attempt to redress the asymmetry of the doctor–patient relationship by institutionalising shared decision-making. Also, the pressure of economic rationing in hospitals quickly leads to the abandonment of the unspecified requirements of psycho-social medicine, which, beyond the organ medicine, wishes to take into account the importance of the 'lifeworld' for pathogenesis and salutogenesis. Extensive doctor–patient discussions are not seen as a medical priority, and, indeed, if they are classed as a routine case, patients will hardly get to see a doctor, because the decisions can be made on the basis of the file documentation.

By using the degrees of freedom the organisation allows, due to its own operative closure, medicine reproduces its own orientation. The fewer physicians who are on duty can maintain a presence by delegating medical controls to the nursing staff, who now have to decide when to call the doctor, the more technology can be deployed which in turn offers arguments for more medical expertise.

Although doctors have suffered a real loss of power and influence with regard to hospital management (cf. Hafferty and Light 1995), their position within medicine is reified with their withdrawal to the role as medical expert. This becomes plain with the requirement for increased reflection of the treatment processes. It is not only necessary to overcome diagnostic uncertainties (Fox 1969) and the problem of therapeutically generated artefacts (Wagner 1995). The speeding-up of processes call for gap management, that is deciding where gaps can be taken into account and how the associated risks can be controlled. At the same time, the settlement modalities of the DRG system generate a new complexity. Only a real medical expert will be able to decode the many layers of medical documentation, including its errors, and to reconstruct the key treatment events behind the various deliberate administrative obfuscations that arise as an answer to the constraints of the increasingly visible economic and legal contextures.

Due to a further 'Taylorisation' of their work, doctors may lose control over the hospital and the treatment process. But, nevertheless, the doctor remains an essential element in the treatment process, in which decisions often have to be taken on the basis of fragmentary information. In accordance with Freidson (2001), who has meanwhile distanced himself from the earlier 'deprofessionalisation' hypothesis, our results suggest that in the modern hospital the three 'logics' of (organisational) bureaucracy, economics and (medical) professionalism are simultaneously being driven to an extreme. In accordance with the neo-institutionalist stance (cf. Meyer and Rowan 1977), economy, bureaucracy and the medical profession can be regarded as being rather loosely linked. But on a systems-theoretical view, they become at the same time more tight coupled, because the different logics become more reflexive about their own boundaries and their own identity through the communicative demands of the other logics.

Our investigations also indicate another class of changes. Whereas in the first observation period the conflict between medical and economic framing was carried out within the medical team and was copied into the doctoral hierarchy, in the more recent example the conflict of interests is reflected in a network of external and stationary care which extends beyond the hospital.

The conflict between the two orientations is carried out in this case not so much between physicians with differing roles (e.g., with the ward physicians siding more with the patient and the senior physicians representing the organisation), but more as a conflict between different organisations or agents within the health-care system. The external nephrologist transfers a patient to the hospital and sidesteps those responsible for taking a decision to have an expensive investigation carried out at the cost of the hospital.

There are indications here of a possible trend in the response to the tensions arising in such situations. Even though some cases now represent an economic risk for the treating organisation, the doctors are not prepared to dispense with a treatment that is in accordance with the best of their professional knowledge. They then have to decide which aspects of the treatment in a complex case can be delegated to which institutions within the treatment network, or which part of the network should shoulder the economic risk anticipated for these treatment processes.[12]

The process of treating the sick is now associated less with a single organisation and is now negotiated less in the intra-organisational dynamic. Rather, it takes place in a treatment network made up of various organisational and personal units. The importance attached to short hospital stays is sufficient to make cooperation necessary with the external services, general practitioners, hospitals, other clinics and stationary care institutions. Not least, the patients and their relatives are themselves also part of the network, since they are called on to cooperate more in the treatment process, whether in the case, the organisation of funds or the organisation of complaints in order to counter the irregularities in the treatment processes.[13] Whereas the old hospital (acting in an unofficial societal function) had to provide not only diagnosis, isolation and therapy but also palliative and end-of-life care in accordance with social indications, these tasks are now distributed among the organisations and individual actors of the treatment networks.[14]

But why do network arrangements appear so attractive under the given conditions? When are networks an answer to polyphony? Returning to the original position, in the hospital, there are various contradictory and incommensurable logics which have to be brought together in an arrangement. In the old-style bureaucratic hospital, which we still encountered at the start of the longitudinal study, economic and medical aspects were still loosely linked inasmuch as shortage of resources determined the setting of the doctor's work. However, economic considerations had not directly impacted the doctor's actions. This changed with the presentational scope of DRGs made possible by computers. Doctors are required to reflect the economic implications of their daily therapeutic and diagnostic decisions. Since medical demands have to be fulfilled and medical failings can have legal consequences, the task faced by doctors resembles the squaring of the circle. Incommensurabilities can no longer simply be ignored but have to be processed simultaneously. As Teubner shows, at this point 'hybrid arrangements' such as networks become interesting.

> [C]ertain economic developments expose actors to a 'double-bind' situation, which they react to with the aid of an internally contradictory network structure. The double-bind situation typical for networks arises where: (1) The social environment makes ambivalent, contradictory or paradoxical demands of business entities which they must respond to; (2) such demands are so central to business survival that they cannot be simply ignored, and (3), their explicit thematization is highly problematical. The institutional answer to these problems is neither contract nor organization, but hybrid network, since this construct allows for the

transformation of external incompatibilities into internally manageable contradictions. [...] In more detail: Hybrid constructions within the triangle of contract, organization and network, facilitate escape from the double-bind situation. They constitute institutional arrangements that make network logic, as opposed to simple contractual or organizational logic, resistant to contradictory social environmental demands. More precisely, hybrids react to paradoxical situations (in their broadest sense) that threaten the operational capacities of actors. [...] Generally-speaking, there are two modes of escape from such imbroglios. The one is repressive, suppressing contradictions by admitting only one of the contradictory instructions and dismissing the other. The other is constructive, seeking to make paradoxes fruitful, to the degree that it establishes a more complex representation of the world.

(Teubner 2006: 12 f.)

The admission of Herr Spondel presented here gives an idea of how these processes can be shaped as contradictory units. The ward physician used the term 'MCA' to refer to the intervention by the external nephrologist into hospital routines which allowed a treatment process that would not otherwise have been possible under the economic logic of the hospitals themselves but that then, by means of a successful 'control test' of the network partner, was able to pave the way for the medical logic of action.[15]

In Luhmann's terminology, the interaction via the treatment network circumvents the organisation to the benefits of the medicine. To quote Teubner once more, '[h]ybrid networks, in this case, appear as manna from heaven, being exactly tailored to bridge multiple contradictory rationalities. They facilitate mutual interference between rationalities without the imposition of hierarchical order' (Teubner 2006: 21).

Regarding a class of observations characterised by the fact that ward doctors consult with other hospitals, care institutions and general practitioners about further proceedings for their patients, this indicates a possible feature of future treatment processes. In treatment networks, the social skills of the doctors were then no longer limited to coping with the situation within the meeting space of their organisation. It would no longer be sufficient to develop a practical feeling for relevances, power struggles and knowledge structures in their organisation. The challenge will be to function in networks, that is, to cope with external control attempts and conversely to exercise control on the partners in the network. The same now also applies for patients and their relatives, who can no longer rely on certainties (also these were only in the form of reliable hierarchical relationships) but must see themselves as an active component of the treatment network and the associated negotiation processes. The uncoupling is now not only (as described by the neo-institutionalists) between the individual spheres within an organisation but takes place in a distributed network of autonomous organisations, with the DRG technology playing a key role in brokering these processes.

DRGs represent in this sense 'leaky black boxes' or 'knowledge objects' (Lowe 2001) around which the networks organise themselves.

In view of the accelerated processes, medical expertise will become even more important under the future conditions, and this is succinctly expressed in the chief physician's statement on medical elegance already documented: 'Do not make things complicated, but think complexly.' This leads to increasing mutual demands between the partners in the treatment network concerning the processing of complexity, the reflection of medicine and resource deployment. In the medium term, this could lead to the economic paradoxical situation that a more economically driven medicine will only come at the price of more expensive expertise.

Notes

1 In the field-observation period of three to twelve weeks' duration, individual treatments were documented synchronously with or near to the process activities during which the actors involved were followed by the observer, who took hand-written notes (cf. Vogd, 2005).
2 With thanks to the Deutsche Forschungsgemeinschaft (German Research Foundation) for financing the follow-up study.
3 I use the concept of frame here after Gregory Bateson (1972). He observed in his studies of play of animals that in different contexts the same behaviour can have very different meanings. In contrast to the frame analysis of Erving Goffman (1986), we concentrate more on the original intention of Bateson and view framing as a collectively created process which in its dynamic goes far beyond the presentation of a social identity. Whether play or seriousness is involved can no longer be viewed as the framing of an individual actor.
4 The concept of polycontexturality and polyphony has similarities to the 'institutional logics' approach (cf. Thornton *et al.* 2012).
5 Trust here is not based on knowledge or norms but appears as a necessary and sensible reduction of complexity (cf. Luhmann 2000c).
6 After Luhmann, codes are limited abstractions, which only apply if the communication chooses their field of application. It is not a matter of truth, right or property in every situation (Luhmann 1986: 79). As Günther Ortmann puts it: 'Actions, operations, payments, transactions, decisions, and communications are by nature ambiguous […] and that seems to me to mean that there can be no distinct economic, legal or political actions, except in the sense that in one or the other context the economic, legal or political aspect is clearly dominant' (2003: 242).
7 For an English introduction to documentary method, see Bohnsack, Pfaff and Weller (Bohnsack *et al.* 2010).
8 For details and further case contrasts, see Vogd (2006).
9 In particular, Wagner (1995) has pointed out that modern medicine can only work well under the current conditions if its decisions also take into account the effects, disturbances, false diagnoses and artefacts which it has produced itself.
10 For example, Tuesday, 3 April 2001, 11.10 a.m.: Chief physician: It is important to do that as thoroughly as possible ... now clarify the vascular disease ... then the thyroid gland ... and if we don't manage to do it here, then write in the letter that the general practitioner can work through it.
11 Certain groups of patients may receive preferential non-medical services in the Organisation Hospital (cf. the chapter on the distinction between privately insured patients and those with standard health insurance in Vogd 2006).

12 According to an estimate in the Deutsche Ärzteblatt, the diagnosis-related groups catalogue in 2005 only covered 50 per cent of the costs for long-stay patients (Billing 2005).
13 This could cast a different light on the prevalence of litigation in America, which can be interpreted as an attempt to introduce control within networks where each party attempts to reach a balance between identity and control.
14 For details of the situation in the USA, see Scott *et al.* (2000).
15 Here in reference to the problem of identity and control and the network theory of Harrison White (1992, 2008).

References

Bateson, G. (1972) *Steps to an Ecology of Mind: Collected Essays in Anthropology, Psychiatry, Evolution and Epistemology*, Aylesbury: Intertext.

Berg, M. (1996) 'Practices of Reading and Writing: The Constitutive Role of the Patient Record in Medical Work', *Sociology of Health and Illness*, 18 (4): 499–524.

Billing, A. (2005) 'Fallpauschalensystem: Problem Schwerstkranke', *Deutsches Ärzteblatt*, 102 (33): A-2214.

Bohnsack, R. (2001) 'Typenbildung, Generalisierung und komparative Analyse. Grundprinzipien der dokumentarischen Methode', in R. Bohnsack, I. Nentwig-Gesemann and A.-M. Nohl (eds.), *Die dokumentarische Methode und ihre Forschungspraxis*, Opladen: Leske und Budrich.

——(2003a) 'Dokumentarische Methode und sozialwissenschaftliche Hermeneutik', *Zeitschrift für Erziehungswissenschaft*, 6 (4): 550–70.

——(2003b) *Rekonstruktive Sozialforschung: Einführung in qualitative Methoden*, Opladen: UTB.

Bohnsack, R., N. Pfaff and W. Weller (2010) *Qualitative Analysis and Documentary Method in International Educational Research*, Opladen and Farmington Hills, Mich.: Verlag Barbara Budrich.

DiMaggio, P. J. and W. W. Powell (1991) 'The Iron Cage Revisited: Institutional Isomorphism and Collective Rationality in Organizational Fields', in W. W. Powell and P. J. DiMaggio (eds.), *The New Institutionalism in Organizational Analysis*, Chicago, Ill.: University of Chicago Press, pp. 41–62.

Foucault, M. (2003) *The Birth of the Clinic: An Archeology of Medical Perception*, London and New York: Routledge.

Fox, R. (1969) 'Training for Uncertainty', in R. K. Merton, G. G. Reader and P. L. Kendal (eds.), *The Student Physician: Intruductory Studies in the Sociology of Medical Education*, Cambridge, Mass.: Harvard University Press, pp. 207–41.

Freidson, E. (1970) *Professional Dominance: The Social Structure of Medical Care*, New York: Atherton Press.

——(1975) *Doctoring Together: A Study of Professional Social Control*, New York: Elsevier.

——(2001) *Professionalism: The Third Logic*, Cambridge: Polity Press.

Goffman, E. (1986) *Frame Analysis: An Essay on the Organization of Experience*, Boston, Mass.: Northeastern University Press.

Hafferty, F. W. and D. W. Light (1995) 'Professional Dynamics and the Changing Nature of Medical Work', *Journal of Health and Social Behavior*, 36: 132–53.

Jachertz, N. (2004) '58 Bayerischer Ärztetag: Bürokratie überwuchert den Arztberuf', *Deutsches Ärzteblatt*, 101 (42): A 2787.

Linczak, G., A. Tempka and N. Haas (2003) 'Verwaltungsaufwand: Entlastung der knappen Ressource Arzt', *Deutsches Ärzteblatt*, 100 (40): A 2563–6.

Lowe, A. (2001) 'Casemix Accounting Systems and Medical Coding: Organisational Actors Balanced on "Leaky Black Boxes"', *Journal of Organizational Change Management*, 14 (1): 79–100.

Luhmann, N. (1986) *Ökologische Kommunikation: Kann die moderne Gesellschaft sich auf ökologische Gefährdungen einstellen?*, Opladen: Westdeutscher Verlag.

——(2000a) *Die Politik der Gesellschaft*, Frankfurt: Suhrkamp.

——(2000b) *Organisation und Entscheidung*, Opladen: Westdeutscher Verlag.

——(2000c) *Vertrauen: Ein Mechanismus der Reduktion sozialer Komplexität*, Stuttgart: Lucius & Lucius.

Meyer, J. W. and B. Rowan (1977) 'Institutionalized Organizations: Formal Structures as Myth and Ceremony', *American Journal of Sociology*, 83 (2): 233–63.

Ortmann, G. (2003) *Organisation und Welterschließung: Dekonstruktionen*, Wiesbaden: Westdeutscher Verlag.

Parsons, T. (1951) *The Social System*, London: Routledge & Kegan Paul.

Power, M. (1997) *The Audit Society: Rituals of Verification*, Oxford: Oxford University Press.

Scott, W. R., M. Ruef, P. J. Mendel and C. R. Caronna (2000) *Institutional Change and Healthcare Organizations: From Professional Dominance to Managed Care*, Chicago, Ill.: University of Chicago Press.

Strauss, A., L. Schatzman, D. Ehrlich, R. Bucher and M. Sabshin (1963) 'The Hospital and Its Negotiated Order', in E. Freidson (ed.), *The Hospital in Modern Society*, London: Free Press, pp. 147–69.

Teubner, G. (2006) 'Coincidentia Oppositorum: Hybrid Networks Beyond Contract and Organization', in R. Grodon and M. Horwitz (eds.), *Festschrift in Honour of Lawrence Friedman*, Palo Alto, Calif.: Stanford University Press, pp. 3–30.

Thornton, P. H., W. Ocasio and M. Lounsbury (2012) *The Institutional Logics Perspective: A New Approach to Culture, Structure and Process*, Oxford: Oxford University Press.

Vogd, W. (2002) 'Professionalisierungsschub oder Auflösung ärztlicher Autonomie. Die Bedeutung von Evidence Based Medicine und der neuen funktionalen Eliten in der Medizin aus system- und interaktionstheoretischer Perspektive', *Zeitschrift für Soziologie*, 31 (4): 294–315.

——(2004a) 'Ärztliche Entscheidungsfindung im Krankenhaus bei komplexer Fallproblematik im Spannungsfeld von Patienteninteressen und administrativ-organisatorischen Bedingungen', *Zeitschrift für Soziologie*, 33 (4): 26–47.

——(2004b) *Ärztliche Entscheidungsprozesse des Krankenhauses im Spannungsfeld von System- und Zweckrationalität: Eine qualitativ rekonstruktive Studie*, Berlin: VWF.

——(2004c) 'Entscheidung und Karriere: Organisationssoziologische Betrachtungen zu den Geschehnissen einer psychosomatischen Abteilung', *Soziale Welt*, 55 (3): 283–300.

——(2005) 'Teilnehmende Beobachtung', in S.-U. Schmitz and K. Schubert (eds.), *Einführung in die Politische Theorie und Methodenlehre*, Opladen: Verlag Barbara Budrich.

——(2006) *Die Organisation Krankenhaus im Wandel: Eine dokumentarische Evaluation aus Perspektive der ärztlichen Akteure*, Bern: Huber Verlag.

——(2011) *Systemtheorie und rekonstruktive Sozialforschung: Eine Brücke*, 2nd edn, Opladen: Verlag Barbara Budrich.

Wagner, G. (1995) 'Die Modernisierung der modernen Medizin. Die "epistemiologische Krise" der Intensivmedizin als ein Beispiel reflexiver Verwissenschaftlichung', *Soziale Welt*, 46 (3): 266–81.

White, H. C. (1992) *Identity and Control: A Structural Theory of Social Action*. Princeton, NJ: Princeton University Press.

——(2008) *Identity and Control: How Social Formations Arise*, Princeton, NJ: Princeton University Press.

6 Hospital management
Between medical professionalism and financial pressure

Till Jansen and Sarah Poranzke

Introduction

Multiple, and often diverse, expectations and constraints are placed on doctors by the hospital's management, regulatory agencies and patients (Zuger 2004). In times of ongoing health-care reforms, competition has entered the hospital sector followed by a growing focus by management on hospital administration (Pollitt 1990; Mo 2008). The financial principle is very simple: patient care has to be performed profitably in order keep the hospital competitive in the market. This financial pressure does not necessarily occur on a daily basis because day-to-day medical work is normally driven by medical professionalism (Dopson 1996). In fact, the financial principle may even conflict with the concept of medical autonomy and thus has met resistance among doctors (Harrison and Pollitt 1994). This problem brings daily pressure not only within the departments but also, more so perhaps, at the top. Thus, the position of clinical directors is probably the most interesting where managing different logics is concerned.

From a systems-theory perspective, this conflict can be regarded as a conflict between a medical and an economic contexture. On the one hand, hospitals are organisations that draw from the medical contexture. They apply the code of healthy and sick and strive to produce health. But hospitals are also subject to the economic code. Their communication is observed and has to be observed in reference to the medium of money and the possibility of payment or non-payment in reference to diagnosis and treatment (Vogd 2004). This leads to the question of how organisational communication responds to this problem.

Although this question has been subject to research from different perspectives (Thorne 1997; Gurthrie 1999; Hoff 1999a, 2001; Kitchener 2000; Llewellyn 2001; Witman *et al.* 2011), including that of the perspective of systems theory (Vogd 2004, 2006), the heads of clinical departments have rarely been the focus of attention. Their role has often been described as problematic. Yet the question of how communication here responds to the challenges of conflicting logics has not been addressed.

Our study targets this conflict on the level of the position of clinical directors. Drawing from systems theory, we assumed that organisational practice has a logic of its own that is neither here nor there but rather provides a means of structural coupling for medicine and economy. We have looked at the organisational practice at the level of clinical directors in a qualitative study and reconstructed three different types of related practices.

The chapter first deals with the position of clinical directors in the realms of economic and medical logic. We elaborate on this in the following section using Niklas Luhmann's systems theory and the multi-valued logic of Gotthard Günther. Last, we discuss the design of our empirical study and our findings, comprising three types of logic that lie between economy and medicine.

Clinical directors: between financial needs and medical professionalism

The position of clinical directors lies between economy and the world of the medical profession. On the one hand, it is a medical position, and, on the other hand, it is an administrative position that encompasses the responsibility for the financial success of the department. This conflict between medicine and financial needs is well known in organisational science (Dawson *et al.* 1995; Harrison and Miller 1999; Forbes 2004; Kippist and Fitzgerald 2009).

Nevertheless, the situation of clinical directors varies not only historically but also from one health-care system to another. Clinical directors choose to occupy these positions in different ways and to carve out different careers in them. In many Western countries – and also in the German case we study – clinical directors are doctors first. They have primarily been socialised within the medical profession and thus are used to self-regulation and clinical autonomy (Schultz and Harrison 1986) in performing the primary duty of the profession: patient care. The profession regulates itself by rules of seniority and a professional hierarchy (Witman 2011). Those with the most experience, who excel in science and the practical side of their calling, form the top of the professional hierarchy: they become clinical directors. Chiefs, and thus clinical directors, used to be nominated for this position based on their distinguished medical achievements. They are, therefore, bound to the rules of their profession, as it is the profession that legitimates them.

However, the position of clinical director immediately requires actions that are not covered by the rules of the profession and even collide in many respects with these rules. As soon as doctors become chiefs of departments, they also assume a managerial role and hence become responsible for the financial success – or at least the survival – of their department.

The literature usually addresses this conflict as a problem of conflicting roles, regarded as an internal conflict within the person (Hoff 1999b; Kitchener 2000; Kippist and Fitzgerald 2009). With terms such as two-way window (Llewellyn 2001), hybrid role (Fitzgerald 1994; Kitchener 2000) and double agent (Shortell *et al.* 1998), the situation of the internal conflict of doctors in management has been analysed.

The clinical director is a person who is socialised within the medical profession. He has been trained at least a decade just to meet the expectations of colleagues and patients (Witmann *et al.* 2011). Through the so-called 'hidden curriculum' (Hafferty and Franks 1994) obtained through socialisation, doctors internalise the professional and collegial norms, manners and power relations. Someone who becomes a clinical director of a department such as surgery, cardiology or any other medical speciality will most probably meet the expectations of their profession better than many other colleagues (Thorne 1997).

Paradoxically, the position of a clinical director is awarded to a doctor with outstanding medical achievements who is deeply rooted in the profession and the profession's values. Nevertheless, once they become a clinical director, the time they spends on clinical work diminishes, and the time and effort dedicated to the financial dimension of their function increases. In order to fulfil the organisational needs of the hospital and their department respectively, they have to be open to economic arguments while also maintaining a professional identity by practising medicine in order to maintain their unique value (Hoff 1999a, 1999b), the collegiality and the autonomy of the profession (Thorne 1997).

This analysis is correct up to a point. However, the concept of the two-way window does not fully explain the underlying conflict because the problem is described as resulting from a conflict between the professional socialisation (Fawcett 1988; Hoff 1999b; Schäfer 2002) of doctors and their prospective duties when nominated for the functional position of the clinical director. If this were the scope of the problem, it could be resolved simply by choosing managers rather than doctors to be clinical directors. This is not the case, however. The problem would simply shift within the organisation and would quite possibly result in a conflict between the senior physicians and clinical directors because the underlying conflict must be regarded as an organisational conflict. It results from the fact that hospitals are, on the one hand, companies that have to work according to economic standards and, on the other, medical institutions that work according to the rules of the medical profession. The underlying problem is thus a problem on a much larger scale than a role conflict. It is a structural problem of the hospital organisation caught between the different logics of society (Luhmann 1988, 2005).

The hospital: polycontexturality and clinical directors

The scope of this problem may be best described using Niklas Luhmann's systems theory. Luhmann regards organisations as decision-making systems that couple different functional systems. Hospitals, for example, couple medicine and economy; other systems, such as politics or education, also combine economics with the discipline (Knudsen 2007; Vogd 2011b). Thus, they are confronted with the specific code and media that are used by each functional system. The economic functional system is restricted to the medium of money and the financial results respectively. Its only form of communication is the flow of money. The world, from an economic point of view, is therefore limited to scarce resources and to markets that handle these resources (Luhmann 1988). No other form of observation is possible for a function system. In contrast, the medical-function system deals with sick bodies and develops possible treatments. It uses the code healthy/sick within its communication system (Luhmann 2005).

Hospitals must be regarded separately from these function systems. They are neither part of a medical nor of an economic, or perhaps an administrative, function system. Hospitals are organisations and, as such, observe function systems as part of their environment. They observe developments within markets and new standards in medical treatment (e.g., evidence-based medicine). They observe reforms of the payment system and revisions of ICD-10 code (International Statistical Classification of Diseases and Related Health Problems), and they develop strategies to handle the different expectations of these environments.

Yet, from within the organisation, the function systems are as much within the organisation as they are outside. They appear to be outside, for example, if a new drug has been authorised by the responsible authority or a new DRG standard has been introduced by the ministry. Naturally, these decisions do not take place within the hospital but rather in the environment. But as soon as these decisions have been made, they have a direct impact on the decision-making within the hospital. They constitute an area of conflict that is best described as polycontexturality (Günther 1979): within the organisation there is an economic logic that refers to economic and financial problems, and there is the professional domain of doctors that draws from medicine and science.

The specific logic of the function systems and the media they use (e.g., money, law, politics) determines the decision-making process within the hospital. They appear as separate logical domains that are simultaneously present (Jansen and Vogd 2013). Each decision can be understood as an economic as well as a medical decision. The contextures are co-present within the organisation. Both exist, and both are relevant, but they exist separately as there is no direct connection between them. Thus, a decision may be an economic decision that promises financial success, but it may contradict a sound medical decision. The opposite might also be true: the best treatment from a medical point of view might also be sound from a financial point of view. In any case, *ab ovo*, the relationship between both contextures is not predetermined. While a decision may represent the positive value within one, it may represent a negative or a positive value within the other. Therefore, double binds may occur if a negative value within one contexture implies a negative value within the other (Bateson *et al.* 1956). Thus far, decision-making in hospitals under the described conditions appears to be problematic if not impossible.

Nevertheless, hospitals do work. They are, more or less, in financial and medical terms successful (at least they survive). The success is only possible because most of the decisions made in hospitals are careful arrangements of different contextures. The treatment of patients may thus, at first glance, appear to be only a medical praxis; however, at second glance, it turns out to be a careful arrangement of different contextures (e.g., Vogd 2004, 2006). Treatments are always chosen with regard to medical and financial consequences, with respect to the relevant law and, sometimes, with respect to the patient. Thus, decision-making within organisations may be regarded as arrangements of different contextures.

The position of clinical directors plays an important role in this respect as it is explicitly positioned between the managerial and the medical contexture. Everyone working in a hospital is confronted with different contextures, clinical directors as much as doctors, nurses or the executive board. No one may work within just one reference. Every manager must understand that running a hospital has to do with medicine just as every doctor must understand that his or her decisions have financial/administrative and legal consequences. Yet there is a fundamental difference between the management and doctors on the one hand and clinical directors on the other: the first group has a predominant reference while clinical directors do not. Doctors make medical decisions with regard to other contextures. They have to keep financial/administrative and legal consequences in mind while treating patients. Management makes economic decisions while keeping legal and medical consequences in mind.

In contrast, clinical directors are subject to a clear double bind: they have to ensure good medical standards, and they are accountable for the financial success of their clinic. Consequently, they have to handle both contextures without a clear predominant reference. As elaborated above, their situation is described with concepts such as two-way window (Llewellyn 2001), hybrid role (Kitchener 2000; Kippist and Fitzgerald 2009) and double agent (Shortell *et al.* 1998). They are as much doctors as managers – and, therefore, have an obvious problem with their self-identity. They are neither here nor there.

Given that hospitals work, and they do in most cases, we assume that there must be a logic that is neither one nor the other, but that is a third instance. It has to be a logic that relates the financial needs of the management to the medical needs of the profession. This logic must be regarded as a logic of the organisation. Here, Gotthard Günther (1979) uses the notion of compound contexture, an emerging order in which a third logic produces a stable relationship between the first two (Jansen and Vogd 2013).

Research question, methodology and sampling

The intention of this paper's research was to reconstruct the third logic that couples financial and medical needs. As this logic has to be regarded as a logic of organisational practice, we chose a qualitative approach that could assure access to the implicit knowledge and the social practice of clinical directors.

The research for this paper began in May 2011 and consisted of thirty-two semi-structured interviews at two German university hospitals. The sample covered interviews with thirty clinical directors as well as the CEOs of both hospitals. The clinical directors in equivalent departments of each hospital were selected among surgical and non-surgical departments. All the clinical directors had been in this position for at least two years and thus had had at least two years of relevant management experience in the dual role.

The interviews were framed by a number of core question areas, including their perception of their role within the hospitals, their experiences with the transition from a clinical to a dual role, the challenges they perceived as relevant in their role, the relationship to the hospital's management and their staff and areas of conflict. The interviews were taped, transcribed and translated into English.

The interviews were analysed using the software program MAXQDA. We chose the documentary method as introduced by Bohnsack (Bohnsack *et al.* 2010) as the interpretation methodology with a special focus on contextural analysis (e.g., Vogd 2009, 2010, 2011a). It aims at reconstructing implicit or atheoretical expectations. These are assumed to structure the social praxis of the interviewees. Thus, by reconstructing it, we gain access to the different techniques that are actually used to arrange different contextures.

The analysis starts from the assumption that there are two different levels to be found within the text. The first level is a manifest sense of the text; it is the '*what*' of the text. With Brunsson (2002), it can also be called the talk that exists inside the organisation: everyone has theories about what he does and what is done inside the organisation. Each person's behaviour is constantly observed and interpreted, is subject to recursive sensemaking (Weick 1995) and becomes shaped by it. If we ask someone what is happening inside the organisation at this level, what we get is theories and interpretations of behaviour and communication rather than behaviour and communication itself. Thus, the interviews may not be taken literally as their content is talk rather than action.

Nevertheless, it is possible to get closer to the level of action as the interviewees offer not only a content (what-level) but also a certain structure (how-level). Behaviour and communication are represented in a certain way, and the way they are presented depends on underlying cognitive frames (Goffman 1986) that structure behaviour and communication. This means that we cannot take literally *what* is said but we can take literally *how* it is said. If, for example, a clinical director tells a story about how he confronted the management, we cannot say whether this story is true or not, but we can say that the story as a story works at the level of semantics: it structures the communication. The norm that is presented by telling this story is actually structuring behaviour. We only reach this level of analysis through constant comparative analysis (Glaser and Strauss 1999). By comparing different positive and negative horizons of contrast, we are able to identify the underlying frames.

The aim of the analysis is thus to identify frames that structure communication. These frames control the relationship between the economic and the medical contexture as they determine the structure of organisational practice. And this practice is neither here nor there. It is not an economic practice nor is it a medical practice. Even if on the level of conversation the clinical director may opt purely for one side, the practice always relates to both. Therefore, it has to be understood as the third logic, the contexture that constitutes the compound contexture.

Results

Our findings showed three different types of logic of organisational practice that related the financial requirements of the management and the logic of managerial professionalism. The first, and most probably the most unsuccessful one, tries to include the medical logic into the economic logic. Professional medical autonomy is seen as no longer maintainable. This kind of relating clearly fails as it is confronted with the resistance of the department. Not understanding that medicine works fundamentally differently than economics, the clinical directors working from within this logic have no grasp of the medical work.

The second logic of organisational practice opts for medical professionalism. Clinical directors working within this kind of logic understand themselves clearly as professionals and defend their autonomy against any attempt at managerial control. Yet, concessions are seen as necessary.

The third logic of organisational practice is the most complex. Although it opts primarily for medicine, medicine and the financial needs of the administration are seen as more complex. While in the first two cases, the relationship between economics and medicine are seen in a dualistic way, the relationship between them blurs in the organisational practice of the third type. Financial needs are no longer regarded as given but as to be determined. Financial needs require something more flexible than a unilateral attempt to control. While the first two ways of relating the economic and medical contexture regard them as ontological constructs that cannot be changed, the third way regards them as logical domains that are rather fuzzy and whose relationship to one another is even more blurred.

Type 1: the dominance of financial threats

The first logic of relating medical and economic contexture regards the relationship as a unilateral attempt to control: financial needs dictate to medicine what has to be done. Furthermore, it opts for the side of the management: the function of the clinical director is to subordinate medical autonomy to economics. Clinical directors working within this logic appear to be rather tragic figures. Trained and socialised as doctors, they have subordinated themselves to management. As such, they are broken professionals, no longer doctors, but neither will they ever become managers:

> We find ourselves in a situation where somebody else is dictating the rhythm of our orchestra. Well, of course, you can argue with that or you can become cynical about it. Or you can accommodate yourself to it. But you have to accept it because it is a fact. In today's hospitals it is the management that directs the orchestra.

The rhythm of the hospital is dictated by the executive board. This metaphor makes clear that the interviewee regards the professional autonomy of the doctors as overruled – at least in his case. He has to adapt to the economic logic, to the rhythms of economy, if he wants to do his job as clinical director. Yet, this is not done easily. It appears that the clinical director is unable to 'feel' the new rhythm he expects himself to adapt to. In the end, he is separate from management rather than a part of it.

> They [hospital management] do not intervene in the day-to-day business of my clinic. I wouldn't even say that they try to run my department. It is the scope of what I can actually decide. Nowadays you are so limited in what you can do by what is set as condition.

The clinical director becomes a simple executor in this interpretation. He is nothing more than a dogsbody to the management having lost all of his former professional autonomy. He is not a *Chefarzt* any longer but only a subordinate to the management.

Even though this type of clinical director is willing to accept the role as subordinate, the dominance of the economical contexture becomes strangely threatening:

> He [the CEO] can take away beds; he can take away my staff. And he is constantly using that as a tool of pressure – permanently. As clinical directors, we have to argue and fight the whole time for the opportunity to achieve our goals – the goals that he has set. Isn't that a paradox? I have to fight for the resources to be able to even try to achieve my goals. I do not get what I need in order to fulfil my goals. It is like I have to fight for the right to achieve the goals that they [the hospital management] set.

In this excerpt, the economic contexture becomes a threat, even though the interviewee is ready to comply with it. He does not understand why he has to fight for his own resources as he assumes that those should be given to him. Bowing to management, reducing oneself to the function of executor, should be sufficient from his point of view. Accepting the aims given by the management should imply getting the resources for it. Yet he still has to fight for the resources he needs to fulfil this function. This shows clearly that it is not sufficient to discard one's autonomy and that it is not even very helpful to do so. Thus, the economic contexture is strangely alien for him.

On the other hand, the medical contexture is threatening, too. His former colleagues are becoming more and more opaque:

> I am pretty sure that there are better ways of doing it than what I am doing it right now. I use as an excuse that at the beginning of a new role you are generally nervous about mistakes. You do not have the sovereignty to know if mistakes happen purely because mistakes happen or if they happen because you are not accepted as the leader. You have to be an authentic leader. I mean you cannot just sit there in your office and send your orders in an email once or twice a week. It doesn't work that way – people don't take you seriously if you are not out there. If you work in a hospital where what we do is treating patients, you always find yourself in a situation that I used to call 'just a heartbeat from disaster'. It might sound a little pathetic; not every patient has a life-threatening condition, of course. But definitely I cannot just do some organizational bits and pieces here and calculate the mistakes that they make and then when the numbers are too high change some other bits and pieces there and once we achieve 10% we all live happily ever after.

This excerpt shows that the interviewed clinical director has not brought his situation under control. He is new to his job and speaks of newbies as 'generally nervous' and lacking the 'sovereignty' to handle the uncertainties that come with his position, feeling that he is always 'one heartbeat from disaster'. This leads to a situation in which he loses contact with his own department and is never sure whether mistakes in the department happen coincidentally or they are the result of resentment and disobedience within the department. His medical colleagues thus become a black box to him, a black box he has to confront as he cannot only 'sit in your office and sent your orders once or twice a week'. He expects himself to be an authentic leader, yet being with his colleagues means being 'out there' in a situation of uncertainty. Consequently, the purely administrative side of his job becomes a kind of retreat for him. The 'organizational bits and pieces' in his office appear as a non-threatening horizon of comparison. Inside this office, everything is under control while 'out there' it's always 'one heartbeat from disaster'.

Thus, leadership within the department becomes something clinical directors of this type wish to reduce to a purely administrative job:

> I thought I would have more time to develop concepts and dedicate time to my leadership. In fact, I have to spend 50% of my time on clinical work. That is way too much. I enjoy it of course, and I wouldn't really

want to miss it. But, in fact, it is time that I lose for leading the department as a manager. But I guess in no way I could neglect clinical work totally, it would mean that I lose touch with [what] we do.

Spending half of his time for clinical work is presented in this case as problematic in leading the department. It becomes clear that the interviewee does not regard medical work as part of management. ('It [medical work] is time that I lose for leading the department as a manager.') The work of a clinical director is conceptualised as purely administrative. Involvement in actual treatment of patients is only necessary in order not to lose touch with the subject of this administrative work.

Comparing the three different passages it becomes clear that the clinical directors of this type are not at home in any of the two contextures. They are neither comfortable with the financial pressure of the management (passage 1), nor are they comfortable as practitioners of medicine. They are not doctors any more (passage 2 and passage 3). Rather, they see their own position somewhere in between, in a rather theoretical domain of administrative and conceptual work. This theoretical domain has to be seen as the third contexture, connecting economics and medicine, constructing the compound contexture of medicine, economics and the practice of managing both. Yet, as the first contextures prove to be a threat to the third, it becomes obvious that the arrangement fails. Both contextures are related to one another in a way that makes a stable coupling impossible. The medical contexture cannot be fully controlled by financial needs. The attempt fails; and the failure of the single clinical directors is just an expression of this failure.

Type 2: defending medicine

The second type is similar in some ways to the first type. Like the first case, the economic contexture is regarded as a threat to medicine. The relationship is seen in dual way: either the code of medicine or the code of managerialism is applied. Yet there is a fundamental difference between Type 1 and Type 2. While the first logic opts for managerialism, Type 2 opts for the side of medicine. Accordingly, the professional roles depicted by these clinical directors are fairly simple: they regard themselves as doctors who are committed to their medical goals:

A doctor cannot be the patient's attorney and the attorney of the government or the insurance companies. In fact, that is the role we have nowadays, because politicians like Ulla Schmidt say, 'Everybody gets everything.' But that does not work out.[1]

The passage shows that the interviewee is aware of multiple, often conflicting environmental demands. But he rejects this multitude of demands by taking them *ad absurdum* and making a caricature of the Ministry of

Health. Rejecting the whole concept of different legitimate demands, he acknowledges one logic, the logic of medical professionalism.

Management is also regarded as restricted to one contexture, but it is another one:

> I consider the relationship to the management of this hospital far from constructive. They [executive committee] have certain demands that might make sense from their perspective, e.g., a hospital is a company that has to produce profits. However, that is incompatible with my medical goals, especially in the long run.

The interviewee opens a dichotomy in this passage. On the one side ('their perspective'), there is the executive committee of the hospital that has to produce profit. The executive committee thus represents economic logic, the pursuit of financial needs. On the other side ('my medical goals') are the doctors who represent the medical contexture. Both contextures are regarded as belonging to one position within the hospital, but they contradict each other as medicine and economics are regarded as conflicting ('the relationship is far from constructive').

This means, first of all, that management is something akin to the natural enemy of all doctors and medical directors (who are only doctors themselves). While management tries to maximise profit, the medical staff is committed to medical aims. The relationship between the clinical director and management is therefore regarded as an open conflict. There is no instance of mediation, no polyvalence, no translation possible between the two of them. There is just an economic contexture (represented by management) and a medical contexture (represented by the medical staff) that clash and fight for dominance. The degree to which this clash is fundamental is shown by the following excerpt by a young clinical director:

> I am still in the comfortable situation that I can always say – if I should think that their financial goals threaten my medical goals – I [will] quit and go somewhere else. Of course, they reply that somewhere else is just the same … but I would take that chance. You have to be consistent.

The conflict between the medical and the economic contexture becomes an existential dimension in this excerpt because it is regarded as a personal struggle of the clinical director. The conflict is not just a role conflict, the result of a specific functional role, management's economic pressure is more a threat to the personal identity of the interviewee. It is not his work that is endangered but the whole person to such a degree that the interviewee might even resign if his medical autonomy should be undermined.

Thus, the medical directors create alliances with their colleagues to defend the work of the departments against the management:

INTERVIEWER: OK, I see. There is the relationship with the hospital's management, and you, as the clinical director, understand how the DRG system works. How about your staff? How do you bridge that gap?

INTERVIEWEE: It is pretty simple. Between the senior physicians and me there are no secrets. I tell them about all the conflicts and fights with the hospital's management. If they release any orders, I discuss it transparently with my senior physicians. We do that once a week. What I don't do, or at least try not to do, is to involve the younger colleagues. In our team, 90% of the doctors are still in a very early stage of their career. I want them to learn how to practice medicine. Good medicine. And the rest, don't even bother with it.

The interviewee makes a distinction between the residents and the senior doctors. The task of the latter he sees as protecting the residents against the management. They should live in a kind of protected atmosphere, purely reserved for the medical contexture. There they are expected to learn their profession thoroughly while not concerning themselves with managerial consequences.

The medical director thus regards himself not as positioned between management and the department but belonging to his department. The senior doctors are regarded as colleagues. He regards them as his equals, not as his staff. His position is not an interface but some kind of barricade, protecting the civilised regions of medicine from the barbarian hordes without that are permanently threatening medical autonomy with a vast arsenal of benchmarks, calculations and PowerPoint presentations.

Sometimes management is even able to break down the barriers and invade the secure territory inhabited by the residents:

INTERVIEWEE: There are these mandatory classes for all the young fellow doctors. There they try educating them that there are certain treatments that have to be done in-patient. And that – of course they don't say that explicitly we have to make things up that we can treat. They allude to it. For example, certain drugs should always be given i.v. Why? It is a justification for in-patient treatment – bullshit I say.

INTERVIEWER: And what do you tell your fellows after such classes?

INTERVIEWEE: We can talk about all that. And it is important that I tell them that I don't support that. I am in charge, and if I say we don't do that here, we simply don't.

Management organises trainings for the residents of the hospital. In these trainings, the financial dimension of the medical work is reflected and the residents receive instructions to make their medical decision-making managerially more efficient. The clinical director tries to undermine the effect of these trainings. Afterwards, he talks with his residents and tells them that he himself does not approve of the suggested strategies.

Thus, every attempt by management to break the clear-cut line between medicine and economy is undermined this type of clinical director. Even if management manages to break down the barrier between management and department and tries to expand the economical contexture to the work of the (protected) residents, the clinical director works in the opposite direction: the broken boundary is repaired or set up anew. The economic contexture is driven out of the medical sphere again.

Interestingly, this type of strategy by clinical directors is limited. As radically as it may be pursued and advocated, it is not possible to separate entirely the medical and economic contexture and keep the financial dimension out of medical work. This is clear enough to those who try; the work of a clinical director is always a kind of compromise:

INTERVIEWEE: In a situation where you see yourself confronted with financial guidelines that you cannot fulfil with your medical way of thinking, of course you start to bend. That is the chicanery.
INTERVIEWER: In which direction are you 'bending'?
INTERVIEWEE: Well, currently I would say, and as I am still young and have plenty of opportunities to go somewhere else, I do not compromise at all. I mean, generally I don't.

Thus, the Type 2 clinical directors try to draw a clean line between medicine and economy while clearly positioning themselves on the medical side. They regard themselves as doctors and nothing else. Their function as clinical director is understood as some kind of border guard: they protect their department from any kind of economic attack by the management. On the practical level, the economic contexture is always there, never to be neglected, but it remains a threat, and a flexible adaptation of both contextures, such as can be seen in Type 3, does not take place. The compound contexture that occurs in Type 3 is more stable than the first case. Yet even the third contexture, the logic of practice of clinical directors, does not manage to integrate economic and medical logic optimally, as we shall see.

Type 3: arranging different worlds

The first, and probably the most important, step towards establishing a stable relationship between medical and managerial contexture is the right definition of clinical work. Clinical directors are the heads of medical departments and are responsible for the medical and financial success of these departments. Nevertheless, the doctors working within these departments are medical staff. They understand themselves exclusively as health-care professionals. Therefore, a definition of good medical work that does not conflict with financial success is necessary. Moreover, a definition is needed that implies a strong coupling between medical and financial success without compromising the integrity of the medical profession. It would not be possible to define medical success as either independent of financial success or subordinate or superordinate to it. These possibilities would either imply the failure of any attempt of financial control or resistance from the medical staff in order to protect their professional autonomy.

Clinical directors respond to this problem by the construction of an implication: medical success is regarded as something that inevitably implies financial success:

> As chief you want things to be done the way you think they have to be done. And you want to organize medicine the way you think it is best for the patient. Needless to say, a high level of acceptance and reputation in the region to attract a high number of patients is what you are aiming to achieve. It is eventually the high inflow of patients that indicates your acceptance in the region.

The interviewee constructs an implication between medical and economic contexture, but not in the sense of Type 1 and Type 2 clinical directors. Rather than stating that economic pressure forces medicine to do what is financially sound, financial success is seen as the result of good medical practice.

This implication maintains the autonomy of the medical practice to a high degree while not neglecting the importance of the economic contexture. This happens on the explicit level. But, on the implicit level, the reverse argument begins to exert this pressure as financial failure can be regarded as result of medical failure.

What also becomes obvious is that clinical directors of this type also opt for the medical contexture. By constructing financial success as implying good medical practice, the medical contexture is regarded as the primary reference. This becomes even clearer in the following passage:

> I don't have the feeling that they try to sabotage me. But I could clearly use some support and understanding of what I am doing here. They always spam you with multiple unimportant things, and I think that they are better off letting somebody else do it. I am an expensive resource. I have the skills to perform sophisticated surgical procedures that only a few people in Germany can do. And they have nothing better to do but to spam me with all this nonsense. I should be treating patients every minute I am here.

Management does not constrain him in his medical work, the interviewee states. Yet he would like more support to do his regular work, his work as a doctor.

It becomes clear in this passage that Type 3 clinical directors regard themselves as doctors. They draw their authority and their self-esteem from their professionalism. In this regard, they are the exact opposite of Type 2 medical directors who long to do as little medical work as possible – just enough not to lose all contact with the medical contexture. However, Type 3 clinical directors also differ from Type 2 clinical directors. While the latter regard the relationship with their management as a conflict, the first do not. Management could do a better job of supporting them, but they are not some kind of natural enemy. This may at first glance be attributed to the management. But a second look makes it clear that this is not the primary reason. The singular management may make a difference; however, the main difference lies in the attitude towards the managerial dimension of the professional medical work:

> Nowadays, it is all a question of income, and how you can improve it. The problem can be very complex. The reason might be of a structural sort, due to competition, for example, or maybe you have the wrong portfolio. Sometimes it is indeed the incompetence of the chief [clinical director]. If he isn't able to gain acceptance among the patients in the region there might be [good] reason for letting him go. That is how it is. We know that. Nowadays it has to be like that.

A doctor's work has a clear economic dimension. From the perspective of the interviewee this cannot be denied. Thus, there is a clear difference between Type 2 and Type 3 clinical directors. While the first believe that medical professionalism has to be protected from any managerial expectation, the latter knows that this is not possible. Yet there is also a difference between Type 3 and Type 2 clinical directors, as Type 2 clinical directors see the managerial dimension of their work only as pressure from the management. This is something Type 1 and Type 2 have in common: the managerial contexture is something that stays outside their realm, that is not fully understood. It is alien to Type 1 as much as to Type 2 clinical directors. Type 3 clinical directors differ on this point. This becomes clear in the latter part of the excerpt, as the interviewee himself starts to argue from a managerial point of view. He identifies different possible reasons for managerial failure of which only one lies within medical practice.

Type 3 clinical directors are able to work within the economic and medical contexture. This can be used to defend medical autonomy. Yet they also know about the necessity of managing successfully. They therefore recode the medical work from an economic point of view where this is possible. This first means using degrees of freedom in medical professionalism:

> Back then [before the introduction of the DRGs] it was best if a patient with a routine treatment stayed with us as long as possible. For example, a patient with a simple appendix resection or an atheroma usually stayed for approximately fourteen days. Today, this doesn't make any sense: you would have to accept multiple deductions of the reimbursement and you wouldn't want to sacrifice that. I mean, it goes without saying

that we have to refer to the actual payment system and try to align clinical work with it. That does not mean that we'd actually go around with a list and select patients that have to go. If a patient isn't in a condition to be discharged, we do not discharge him. It might occur to you that patients are discharged 'bloody' but that doesn't happen.

While before the DRG reform managerial success meant keeping patients as long as possible, today the opposite is the case. This means that patients are discharged as soon as possible.

This is a very simple practice used by almost every clinical director, even Type 1 clinical directors. It is a direct response to a changed payment system. But in the first two cases this practice is seen as being medically unsound, a contravention of the rules of medical professionalism. Conversely, Type 3 clinical directors see it as adapting to financial needs. They know that the former long hospital stays were as much a product of administrative rules as the new practice and that neither way is better or worse from a medical point of view.

This intimate knowledge that medical and financial needs are strongly interwoven, connected by administrative rules, allows them to handle these rules better. Thus, Type 3 clinical directors are able to develop more elaborate forms of adaptation as they know as much about the degrees of freedom within the DRG system as about medical degrees of freedom. They know that neither the managerial nor the medical contexture nor the relationship between the two is fully determined and use this knowledge in a productive manner:

> I try to explain to my staff that our jobs and salaries are only secure if we make it work. That means we deliver good patient care and at the same time assure appropriate reimbursement by coding the work we do. You can discuss who should be responsible for the coding. The doctor? The medical controlling department? Let me tell you; ideally they do it together. The doctor knows exactly what has been done and the controller knows the tricks of coding. To a certain extent you can explain that to your staff. And they accept it. It is still inconvenient, of course, and they don't like it. But they accept it.

Economic success is said to be the precondition of successful medical work. And to be successful, the interviewee states, the medical work has to be sold in the right way. It has to be coded.

Medical and managerial contextures do not appear fully determined in this excerpt. But while the previous excerpt stressed the possibility of adapting the treatment to managerial needs, this excerpt shows that it is quite possible to adapt medical practice to managerial needs without changing the actual practice. This is done by correctly coding, through selling it the right way, so to speak. Each treatment may be interpreted differently. It may be translated differently into DRGs. And doing this translation in a manner that serves the managerial success of the hospital most becomes part of a doctor's work.

The third type of organisational practice thus recognises that the relationship between medical and managerial contexture is not fully determined and that the contextures themselves are not fully determined either. There is not always a medically correct set of practices. Nor is it clear how a certain medical practice is understood from within the managerial contextures. There are degrees of freedom in either case, and recognising these degrees of freedom makes it possible to play with them and to relate managerial and medical contexture in a dynamic way. In consequence, the emerging compound contexture proves to be the most stable one, able to respond to both primary contextures (medicine and economy) optimally.

Summary and conclusion

We identified three types of organisational practice that responded to the problem of the simultaneous presence of medical and managerial contexture. The first two types regarded contextures as a relatively strict set of rules: one dominates while the other one is subordinated. The first type opts for the side of the financial pressure and tries to make the medical contexture fit. Consequently, the clinical directors operating in this logic lose their autonomy as they lose their medical professionalism; they have neither authority within their department nor a sound foundation from which to oppose hospital management. The result is a less successful practice. The second type opts for the side of the medical contexture and resists the financial pressure exerted by management. The clinical directors thus preserve their professional identity as a zone of autonomy but nevertheless have to make concessions to financial needs. The most complex logic of organisational practice is the third type. Like the second type, the third type opts for the side of medicine, but it regards the economic contexture as less of a threat. From within this logic, medicine and managerialism do not appear to be so strict and mutually exclusive. Rather, degrees of freedom within each contexture are recognised, and the relationship between both is regarded as flexible.

From the perspective of the organisation, the presence of polycontexturality can mean different things. The first two types of organisational practice prove to be insufficiently complex to respond to a situation where two – or more – logics are applied at the same time. They are not able to interweave both logics in a productive way. Rather, they produce conflict – either between the clinical director, the doctors, and the hospital management (Type 1) or between the clinical directors and the hospital management. Only Type 3 organisational practice actually reflects the complexity of a polycontextural society and works with it in a productive manner. Organisational practice thus becomes crucial for the consequences of health care in a polycontextural

world. The ability to shift logics, to apply certain frames in the right situation, to specify and to blur becomes important. The management of a clinical department thus becomes a fuzzy thing. It is a practice that thrives on
ambivalence and a consequent postponing.

On an abstract level, successful management seems to be based on a kind
of deontologised or relativist epistemiology and/or pragmatism. The practice Type 3 clinical directors all had in common was that they did not regard
medical nor financial demands as fixed. Neither the medical nor the economic logic appeared as a fixed set of rules and norms with clear guidelines
for right and wrong, whereas in the case of the first two types, this was the
case. Type 3 provided a more fluid interpretation of sound medical treatment and financial success. Both logics were interpreted as logics, having
relatively clear boundaries but not being determined by these boundaries.
In the first two cases, the boundaries also seemed clear, but, at the same
time, the content also seemed to be fixed. To put it simply: while in the first
two cases there was only one right way to do something, in the last case,
there proved to be multiple ways that were all right to a certain degree but
often also wrong to a certain degree. Nevertheless, this provides freedom of
choice.

Moreover, the first two types tended to confront medical and economic
logic. This is perhaps a direct consequence of conceptualising a logic as
fixed. As soon as a certain medical practice is no longer regarded as contingent – at least to a certain extent – a direct conflict appears when another
logic presents a conflicting demand. If, for example, there appears to be
only one way to deal with a medical problem but there is no choice from
a financial point of view, a direct conflict results. If this conflict is further
conceptualised as not being limited to one, or perhaps only a small number
of cases, it becomes a general conflict between two logics. Consequently, a
clinical director has to choose one side, fighting the other. The interpretation
of Type 3 is less fundamental. It does not confront both logics but rather
interlaces them. This does not mean that they are always compatible – that
is not the case – but it does mean that medical management means to deal
with both logics, always arranging them in a new relationship.

On an empirical level, the preconditions for the third type of practice seem
to be mainly experience. Clinical directors with long experience in their job
tend more towards Type 3 than young clinical directors. This may have to
do with the experience of contingency. Many clinical directors of the third
type did relate stories about times when practices were different – practices
of accounting and medical practices – and it worked out, too. Yet it is difficult to say what was first, the chicken or the egg. First of all, experiences
have to be gained over time. Having only experienced different kinds of
practices does not mean that the actual practices are regarded as contingent.
The change of medical practice can also be interpreted as a result of growing
knowledge. In consequence, the up-to-date practice may appear to be even
more state-of-the-art practice, the best and only way to act. Brunsson has

shown similar processes (2006). Furthermore, Type 3 clinical directors will most probably be more successful in their jobs keeping their posts longer. In fact, one of the Type 2 clinical directors we interviewed has already resigned. Thus, the longer experience of Type 3 clinical directors may be also a result of their staying longer on the job. It does not necessarily mean that Type 1 or 2 clinical directors become Type 3.

The findings of this research are limited to German hospitals. Only two hospitals were examined, so the results may not be regarded as representative for the whole sector. Nevertheless, the various interviews have shown a high degree of theoretical saturation. That said, further research is necessary to obtain more reliable results. A comparison with other health-care systems would be particularly interesting, especially a situation in which a department is led by two directors, one who is primarily responsible for medical issues and the other for managerial issues. It would be interesting to observe how the difference between economic goals and medicine is dealt with here.

Notes

1 Ulla Schmidt is a German politician who was Minister of Health from 2001 to 2009.

References

Bateson, G., D. D. Jackson, J. Haley and J. Weakland (1956) 'Toward a Theory of Schizophrenia', *Behavioral Sciences*, 1 (1): 251–64.
Bohnsack, R. (2003) *Rekonstruktive Sozialforschung: Einführung in qualitative Methoden*, Opladen: Leske + Budrich.
Bohnsack, R. P., N. Pfaff and V. Weller (eds.) (2010) *Qualitative Analysis and Documentary Method in International Educational Research*, Opladen: Budrich.
Brunsson, N. (2002) *The Organization of Hypocrisy: Talk, Decisions and Actions in Organizations*, Copenhagen: Copenhagen Business School Press.
——(2006) *Mechanisms of Hope: Maintaining the Dream of the Rational Organization*, Copenhagen: Copenhagen Business School Press.
Dawson, S., V. Mole, D. Winstanley and J. Sherval (1995) 'Management, Competition and the Professional Practice: Medicine and the Marketplace', *British Journal of Management*, 6 (3): 132–56.
Dopson, S. (1996) 'Doctors in Management: A Challenge to Established Debates', in J. Leopold, M. Hughes and I. Glover (eds.), *Beyond Reason? The National Health Service and Limits of Management*, Aldershot: Avebury, pp. 173–87.
Evers, H. (2009) 'The Documentary Method in Intercultural Research Scenarios', *Forum Qualitative Sozialforschung/Forum: Qualitative Social Research*, 10 (1). Available online at http://nbn-resolving.de/urn:nbn:de:0114-fqs0901478 (accessed 23 June 2014).
Fawcett, T. (1988) 'OPC: Organisational Professional Conflict', *Australian Accountant*, 58 (93) 93.

Fitzgerald, L. (1994) 'Moving Clinicians into Management: A Professional Challenge or Threat?' *Journal of Management in Medicine*, 8 (6): 32–44.

Forbes, T., J. Hallier and L. Kelly (2004) 'Doctors as Managers: Investors and Reluctants in a Dual Role', *Health Services Management Research*, 17 (3): 167–76.

Garfinkel, H. and H. Sacks (1986) 'On Formal Structures of Practical Actions', in Harold Garfinkel (ed.), *Ethnomethodological Studies of Work*, London: Routledge & Kegan Paul, pp. 162–3.

Glaser, B. and A. Strauss (1999) *The Discovery of Grounded Theory: Strategies for Qualitative Research*, New York: Aldine.

Goffman, E. (1986) *Frame Analysis: An Essay on the Organization of Experience*, Boston, Mass.: Northeastern.

Günther, G. (1979) 'Life as Poly-contexturality', in Günther Gotthard (ed.), *Beiträge zur Grundlegung einer operationsfähigen Dialektik*, vol. II: *Wirklichkeit als Poly-Kontexturalität*, Hamburg: Felix Meiner Verlag, pp. 283–307.

Gurthrie, M. B. (1999) 'Challenges in Developing Physician Leadership and Management', *Frontiers of Health Services Management*, 15 (4): 3–26.

Hafferty, F. W. and R. Franks (1994) 'The Hidden Curriculum, Ethics Teaching and the Structure of Medical Education', *Academic Medical*, 69 (11): 861–71.

Harrison, R. and S. Miller (1999) 'The Contribution of Clinical Directors to the Strategic Capability of the Organisation', *British Journal of Management*, 10 (1): 22–39.

Harrison, S. and C. Pollitt (1994) *Controlling Health Professionals: The Future of Work and Organisation in the NHS*, Buckingham: Open University Press.

Hoff, T. (1999a) 'The Paradox of Legitimacy: Physician Executives and the Practice of Medicine', *Health Care Management Review*, 24 (4): 54–64.

——(1999b) 'The Social Organization of Physician-Managers in a Changing HMO', *Work and Occupations*, 26 (3): 324–51.

——(2001) 'Exploring Dual Commitment among Physician Executives in Managed Care', *Journal of Healthcare Management*, 46 (2): 92–111.

Jansen, T. and W. Vogd (2013) 'Polykontexturale Verhältnisse – disjunkte Rationalitäten am Beispiel von Organisationen', Zeitschrift für theoretische Soziologie (ZTS), 1 (2): 82–97.

Kippist, L. and A. Fitzgerald (2009) 'Organisational Professional Conflict and Hybrid Clinical Managers', *Journal of Health Organisation and Management*, 23 (6): 642–55.

Kitchener, M. (2000) 'The Bureaucratization of Professional Roles: The Case of Clinical Directors in UK Hospitals', *Organization*, 7 (1): 129–54.

Knudsen, M. (2007) 'Structural Couplings between Organizations and Function Systems: Looking at Standards in Health Care', *Cybernetics and Human Knowing*, 14 (2–3): 111–31.

Llewellyn, S. (2001) 'Two Way Windows: Clinicians as Medical Managers', *Organization Studies*, 22 (4): 593–623.

Luhmann, N. (1988) *Die Wirtschaft der Gesellschaft*, Frankfurt: Suhrkamp.

——(2005) 'Der medizinische Code', in *Soziologische Aufklärung 5*, VS Verlag für Sozialwissenschaften, pp. 176–88.

Mo, T. (2008) 'Doctors as Managers: Moving towards General Management? The Case of Unitary Management Reform in Norwegian Hospitals', *Journal of Health Organization and Management*, 22 (4): 400–15.

Nassehi, A. (2002) 'Die Organisation der Gesellschaft: Skizze einer Organisationssoziologie in gesellschaftstheoretischer Absicht', in J. Allmendinger and T. Hinz (eds.), *Organizationssoziologie*, Opladen: Westdeutscher Verlag, pp. 443–78.

Pollitt, C. (1990) *Managerialism and the Public Services*, Oxford: Blackwell.

Reed, M. (1996) 'Expert Power and Control in Late Modernity: An Empirical Review and Theoretical Synthesis', *Organization Studies*, 17 (4): 573–97.

Schäfer, W. E., J. L. Park and M. L. Woody (2002) 'Professionalism, Organizational-Professional Conflict and Work Outcomes: A Study of Certified Management Accountants', *Accounting, Auditing and Accountability Journal*, 15 (1): 46–68.

Schultz, R. and S. Harrison (1986) 'Physician Autonomy in the Republic of Germany, Great Britain and the United States', *International Journal of Health Planning and Management*, 1 (5): 335–55.

Shortell, S., T. Water, P. Budetti and K. Clarke (1998) 'Physicians as Double Agents: Maintaining Trust in the Era of Multiple Accountabilities', *Journal of the American Medical Association*, 280 (12): 1102–8.

Thorne, M. L. (1997) 'Being a Clinical Director: First among Equals or Just a Go-Between?', *Health Services Management Research*, 10 (4): 205–15.

Vogd, W. (2004) *Ärztliche Entscheidungsprozesse des Krankenhauses im Spannungsfeld von System- und Zweckrationalität: Eine qualitativ rekonstruktive Studie unter dem besonderen Blickwinkel von Rahmen (frames) und Rahmungsprozessen*, Berlin: Verlag für Wissenschaft und Forschung.

——(2006) *Die Organisation Krankenhaus im Wandel*. Eine dokumentarische Evaluation aus Sicht der ärztlichen Akteure. 1. Aufl. Bern: Huber.

——(2009) *Rekonstruktive Organisationsforschung: Qualitative Methodologie und theoretische Integration – eine Einführung*, Opladen: Budrich.

——(2010) 'Methodologie und Verfahrensweise der dokumentarischen Methode und ihre Kompatibilität zur Systemtheorie', in R. John, A. Henkel and J. Rückert-John (eds.), *Die Methodologien des Systems: Wie kommt man zum Fall und wie dahinter?* Wiesbaden: VS Verlag für Sozialwissenschaften/GWV Fachverlage, pp. 121–40.

——(2011a) *Systemtheorie und rekonstruktive Sozialforschung – eine Brücke*, 2nd edn, Leverkusen: Barbara Budrich.

——(2011b) *Zur Soziologie der organisierten Krankenbehandlung*, Weilerswist: Velbrück.

Waldmann, J. D., H. Smith, J. Hood, and S. J. Pappelbaum (2006) 'Healthcare CEOs and Physicians: Reaching Common Ground', *Journal of Healthcare Management*, 51 (3): 171–84.

Weick, Karl E. (1995) *Sensemaking in Organizations*, Thousand Oaks, Calif.: Sage.

Witmann, Y., G. A. C. Smid, P. L. Meurs and D. Willems (2011) 'Doctor in the Lead: Balancing between Two Worlds', *Organization*, 18 (4): 477–95.

Zuger, A. (2004) 'Dissatisfaction with Medical Practice', *New England Journal of Medicine*, 350 (1): 69–76.

7 Sustainability in integrated-care partnerships

A systems and network theoretical approach for the analysis of cooperation networks

Daniel Lüdecke

Introduction

The general discussion on integrated care sees the (urgent) necessity that organisations in the health and social-care sector in Germany should cooperate and implement integrated care programmes, as support services are highly fragmented and there is a strict separation of supply and care sectors. The care sectors are split into stationary (in-patient) care with services such as hospitals or care and nursing homes; partly stationary care with services such as day care or rehabilitation facilities; and finally the ambulatory sector with many different services such as home care, mobile services, therapists, general practitioners and so on. Then again, the support services are highly specialised in their tasks and offers, so that a comprehensive supply of people in need of care could only be established by the cooperation and integration of the different help providers (integrated-care partnerships) (Bräutigam *et al.* 2005; Dt. Caritasverband 2005; Kurlemann 2010).

Furthermore, an economic necessity to cooperate was established by a new financing and remuneration system within the health-care sector. Since 2004, the costs for medical treatments in German acute hospitals are calculated by classifying patients into groups based on their diagnosis. These so-called diagnosis-related groups (DRGs) indicate the average amount of resources a medical treatment consumes (Herwartz and Strumann 2013; Quentin *et al.* 2013). The former financing system covered the costs of how long a patient stayed in hospital, thus giving fewer incentives to discharge a patient as soon as possible. Now hospital guidelines specify an average hospital stay for patients and leave further treatment to other health-care providers (Glaeske 2002; Stock *et al.* 2005).

Increasing costs and decreasing hospitalisation require network-like cooperations (Vogd 2009a), thus enforcing integrated-care partnerships. The assumption is that a better cooperation leads to faster transitions of patients from one provider to the next and, as a result, to more financial benefits from medical treatments. Each involved organisation has to manage tasks linked between the cooperating organisations to enable trouble-free workflows within this network. However, current studies still outline the deficiency in integrated-care partnerships (Glaeske 2002; Wingenfeld 2002; Bühler 2006; Ommen *et al.* 2007; Heaton *et al.* 2012). The practical implementation of cooperation turns out to be more difficult than anticipated.

Objectives

The assumption made in this chapter is that the process of integrated care is too complex for simplified, rational guidelines. Organisations in general, and this applies to organisations in the health-care and nursing sector, especially to hospitals, can be seen as complex social systems. These systems consist of hardly comprehensible and understandable amounts of relations between elements. This makes it almost impossible to achieve a holistic picture and understanding of all of an organisation's processes. Organisations have their own logic and dynamics.

Referring to Luhmann's systems theory (1984, 1996), society is differentiated into various function systems that operate on the basis of a *mono-contextural* structure due to the binary coding of each system (Luhmann 2005).[1] Yet organisations have to deal with paradoxes (or to use Günther's phrase [1979], with conflicting *contextures*) because they are exposed to different function systems simultaneously (polycontexturality). Typically, organisations then have to transform these paradoxes into decisions to gain capacity to act (Luhmann 2000). In this understanding, organisations can be considered as *polyphonic organisations* (Åkerstrøm Andersen 2003) that behave in a way that lets them appear to be 'irrational' (Brunsson 1985; Weick 1995; Vogd 2008; Brunsson *et al.* 2012).[2] Assuming that organisations' (systems') processes appear as difficult to understand for outside observers, how is cooperation possible? How do network structures emerge, and which factors have an impact on the sustainable structure of cooperation networks?

In this chapter, we want to explore the meaning of *sustainability* in the context of integrated-care partnerships, taking into account polycontextural conditions (Günther 1979). Organisations in the health-care system are confronted with the dilemma of harmonising numerous, possibly conflicting, requirements. For instance, there is the medical system that claims need for a high quality of medical supply and comprehensive patient-centred care. The economic system, however, controls access and distribution of resources (Luhmann 1994). Thus, medical treatment has to be achieved with limited financial resources due to the economic requirements from the DRG system. In such a case, economic demands may work against medical necessities. The medical and economic system both refer to their own contextures that have to be 'balanced', i.e. intermediation contextures emerge that order the relationship between these contextures to gain capacity to act (Kaehr 1993; Jansen and Vogd 2013). In the course of the 'process of organising' (Weick *et al.* 2005), the different contextures are arranged in a way that allows for decision-making. Taking the basic conflict between medical and economic systems into account, the question is which controlling mechanism is applied to arrange these polycontextural conditions.

From a classical point of view, organisations and their structural characteristics can be located on a continuum between hierarchy and market. Decisions made in organisations may refer to authority (hierarchy) or are based on market demands, where 'prices capture all relevant information necessary' for decision-making (Powell 2011: 31). In the past there was a 'professional dominance' (Freidson 2007) in medical care where doctors acted as guarantors in the bureaucratic structures of hospitals. Being autonomous professionals, doctors decided on patients' medical treatment and their hospital discharge. Handling the balance between medical and economic requirements was in the doctors' authority (McKinlay 1977; Freidson 1980; Hafferty and Light 1995). The economic pressure was rather low. Medical care was the dominant contexture. This has recently changed dramatically with the introduction of DRGs. It seems that there has been a shift on the continuum away from hierarchy towards market. The DRG as compensation system can be considered as new arising contexture (assigned to the economic system) with the intention to control the discharge and transition planning in integrated-care partnerships. Hospitals perceive a high pressure to adapt this outside disturbance (Schaeffer and Ewers 2006; Vogd 2012). Specified rates now limit payments for medical treatments. This leads to decreasing hospitalisation, which, in turn, requires hospitals to treat more cases. Limits for payments are installed to counterbalance inappropriate supply (e.g., undersupply) of patients (Quentin *et al.* 2013).

However, if organisations are considered as systems as defined by systems theory, they are assumed to be autonomous in their decision-making. Thus, integrated and patient-centred care cannot be controlled from outside, for instance due to environmental disturbance caused by the DRG system. Powell (2011) argues in a similar way. Organisations behave in a way that can be explained neither by referring to authority (hierarchy) nor by the logic of markets. Moreover, organisations cannot be considered as hybrid composition of hierarchy and market characteristics. Rather, organisations are located in cooperation structures that rely much more on reciprocity, mutual interests and appraisal. Organisational behaviour is much more embedded in social structures, which cannot be sufficiently explained by either formal structures of hierarchy or profit-orientation. Powell suggests calling this control mechanism *networks* (2011). From this perspective, networks appear as independent control mechanism for sustainable, self-organising integrated-care partnerships. The assumption is that networks may work as intermediation contexture that arranges polycontextural conditions (medical and economic contextures). The question is how these networks can effectively carry out control on integrated-care partnerships and keep these relationships stable among conditions of hierarchical and market impacts. Empirical analyses have been conducted to give an insight into the practice of these kinds of cooperation networks.

Theoretical context

Systems theory as theoretical framework for the analysis

Following the idea to construct organisations as social systems, we have to outline to which kind of systems theory these thoughts refer. In this case, we try to build a theoretical framework to analyse the cooperation of organisations by applying the systems theory by Niklas Luhmann (1984, 1996). It is important to point out this reference because there are various developments and offshoots of systems theories that differ noticeable in their core concepts, for instance:

- open systems versus operational closure;[3]
- recursive self-reproduction of structures (autopoiesis);[4]
- action versus communication (or, causality versus complexity).[5]

From the perspective of Luhmann's systems theory, organisations no longer appear as purpose-rational institutions, defined by their members, that pursue their own interests. Rather, organisations are 'purpose-seeking systems' (Luhmann 2000: 165; March and Olsen 1979) that reproduce themselves qua the operation of communication of decisions. On this note, purposes are no longer understood in a context where motives explain the action of members. An organisation evolves independent from its members' purposes.

Organisation as social system

Organisations are social systems of own type and quality (Luhmann 2000; Simon 2007). This is, of course, also true for organisations in the health-care sector such as hospitals, ambulatory care services or care and nursing homes (Grossmann and Scala 2002a). Considering organisations as systems means that concepts of operational closure and complexity or indeterminacy also apply. This raises questions regarding the controlling or steering capabilities of organisations. How is cooperation between and coordination of organisations achieved?

Controlling (or steering) a system

A system always tries to keep its own autopoiesis in progress, which means to survive. The priority of a system lies in the maintenance of its own structures. Exterior exertion of influence on an organisation's progresses and workflows always faces the problem that an organisation simply may not do what people from outside would expect, especially when the influences are regarded as a too intensive disturbance and are incompatible with the organisation's structures. That is why organisations are considered self-logical, having their own dynamics and following their own rules. Taking operational closure seriously means that there are no conjoint binding rules for all organisations which are involved in the integrated care and interface management process (Grossmann and Scala 2002b; Besl 2011). Decisions and routines made in one organisation are not automatically applied to or accepted by other organisations. There is no central instance or authority for controlling (steering) the integrated care and cooperation process. Different organisational structures have to be taken into account.

When an organisation (system) cannot directly control the other organisations (environment), how is cooperation possible? How can mutual attempts of exertion of influence innervate structural changes within organisations and affect their commitment to cooperate? Or, how do systems 'open' themselves for environmental influence although they are operationally closed?

Structural coupling

Operational closure is a prerequisite for the openness of systems in order to identify the system's boundaries: which elements and events belong to the system, which ones to the environment? Operational closure allows a system's state and its operations to be distinguished as opposed to those of the environment. The possibility of clearly identifying the difference between system and environment enables the system to look at specific sections of the environment to handle its complexity and make these environmental structures manageable for own stipulation. This process is called *structural coupling*. Structural coupling explains the mutual dependency and possibility of exertion of influence of two systems or of systems and their environment (Luhmann 1992; Baecker 2001). Although, or better, because systems are operationally closed, they allow themselves to be controlled from other structural coupled systems or by systems in their environment on which they depend. Again, this disturbance stimulates a structural drift, so the coupled system(s) can establish or change certain structures.

With regard to the question how organisations (systems perspective) can cooperate and their workflows be coordinated (network perspective), the concept of structural coupling is helpful in so far as it offers the possibility to combine the systems and network perspectives (Baecker 1997, 2001). Our hypothesis is that sustainability fits into this concept because it refers both to structural changes within organisations (systems perspective) as well as to the conditions of networking of organisations (network perspective).

Sustainability

Sustainability belongs to the common everyday language and is used in many different contexts. This highlights the arbitrariness of this term and points out how difficult it is to find an appropriate conception of sustainability. Furthermore, the discussion about sustainability implies a predictable future: acting sustainably means to gain benefits in the future, for example, having more available resources (Glasby 2002; Wetzel 2005; Harvard Business Manager 2007; Laloe 2007). However, due to the complexity of the interface-management process and the complexity of each involved system (organisation), predictability becomes difficult (Grossmann and Scala 2002b; Simon 2007; Fuchs 2008a). One could say that complexity almost excludes predictability. One aspect seems to be a core aspect of the various sustainability definitions: leaving the future undetermined and, at the same time, ensuring forthcoming possibilities of change and development (Luks 2002).

Such an understanding of sustainability seems paradoxical because it combines *reversibility* (keeping possibilities of structural modifications open) and *irreversibility* (maintaining desired effects) (Fuchs 2008b). While irreversibility can be assigned to *system processes* that are fixed concatenations of occurrences, the sphere of influence, and thus possibilities of controlling systems, rather applies to *system structures*. Structures are characterised by a specific flexibility, allowing miscellaneous occurrences to happen and are also able to manage irritations, which are not yet compatible with their own structures. Hence, sustainability should be applied as 'schematised irritation' to become a successful strategy. In integrated-care partnerships, sustainability means stimulating feedback (resonance) in the networked organisations and thereby mutually stabilising expectations and reliance.

Networks

As said before, each organisation has certain *expectations* of what the other network partners can or should do, and for which tasks oneself is responsible. Networks, however, in a sociological sense, are the attempt to develop, form and control identities and to push through own interests (Baecker 2005; White 2008). The ways in which an organisation can appear, behave and claim its own interests (identity) is influenced and 'limited' by other organisations' attempts of controlling network processes and vice versa. Nevertheless, as mentioned above, attempts of controlling other organisations (systems) are difficult and usually fail. Thus, controlling a network cannot aim at enacting compulsory guidelines organisations have to comply with. Rather, control means to develop expectations and permanently adjust these expectations according to the actual occurrences in networks. This explains what Powell (2011) describes as a basic assumption of network relationships: 'one party is dependent on resources controlled by another' and 'the parties to a network agree to forego [sic] the right to pursue own interests at the expense of others' (Powell 2011: 35). For this reason, *networks* can be considered as another mechanism for controlling partnerships in addition to hierarchical or market structures.

Integrated-care partnerships and sustainability

Being part of a network means to negotiate tasks and obligations with other organisations of this network. What can I expect from others? Which expectations do I have to fulfil to stay in the network? A cooperation network is a fragile structure that requires permanent 'interface management' and perpetual negotiations about the distribution of uprising tasks. Sustainability indicates a *reflection strategy* of organisations (Drucker 2001; Wetzel 2005). In integrated-care partnerships, each party has to become sensitive to observing the difference between self-perception and how others perceive them in the network (feedback, resonance). In essence, *networks* as controlling mechanisms forward the emergence of sustainable, effectively (self-) organised integrated-care partnerships, without the need for hierarchical or market impacts.

However, we have to take into account the increasing economic pressure that lies on health and social-care providers on the one hand as well as the need for patient-centred care on the other hand. The involved parties have to deal with polycontexturality, i.e. in this particular subject the concurrent presence of hierarchic, bureaucratic determination, economic and medical requirements, and find ways to 'incorporate' these demands into the network structures. This means incorporating mentioned demands in their decision-finding to gain capacity to stabilise the network. In this spirit, following the idea of Åkerstrøm Andersen (2008) to consider networks as 'reflexive contracts', networks can be regarded as intermediation contexture that balances the dilemma of medical and economic requirements by reflexive awareness. In the context of integrated-care partnerships, new degrees of freedom arise that ensure professional autonomy of network partners, while at the same time the self-organisation of network relationships is conditioned by mutual observations.

Methods

An appropriate way to set up a sociological research programme that analyses the process of integrated-care partnerships, embedded into a theoretical systems and networks context, is to use *reconstructive* empirical methods. This approach assumes that organisations and the process of integrated care are dynamic subjects that cannot be defined by certain criteria. This can then be used for building hypotheses. An organisation creates its own rules and purposes by itself (Vogd 2009b).

A reconstructive method tries to describe the *self-organisation* of an object of investigation from this object's *self-logical* understanding. The focus lies on the principles of self-organisation not on the subjective meaning of individuals. It is no longer important *what* people might mean or which underlying motifs probably lead to their actions but *how* statements materialise, i.e. which (organisational) structures or framings have an impact on how people talk about specific subjects (Vogd 2010). This approach accommodates for the self-logic and dynamics of organisations, taking into account that a systems-theoretical perspective considers organisations as *polyphonic*, i.e. approves of polycontexturality. In their day-to-day work, people face conflicting needs that have to be transformed into decisions that control their actions (Sadler 2001; Baecker 2002; Kölking 2007). The researcher now has to explore the ways of *decision-finding in organisations*, how it varies depending on the professional contexts and foci of actors in organisations and how actors deal with different perspectives (contextures) in order to come to a decision (Vogd 2008). In the context of reconstructive (organisational) research, the aim is to find these contradictions and the practical implementation of their solutions. This approach is appropriate for analysing organisations as its epistemological foundations are similar to the epistemology of Luhmann's systems theory (Vogd 2009c; Bohnsack 2010).

Documentary method

We follow the suggestions of Vogd (2010) and Bohnsack (2007, 2010) to use the *documentary method* as a qualitative research approach, which seems to be promising and suitable for this purpose. Following this method, the researcher tries to reconstruct the *modus operandi* of (organisational) practice. It is no longer important to look at *why* people act the way they act and to find reasons for their actions. Rather, the question is, *how* social formations emerge (Bohnsack 2007; Vogd 2009b): the focus lies on the process of sense making in organisations (Weick 1995; Weick *et al.* 2005). Especially with regard to the empirical analysis, the documentary method is able to identify the different contextures and give insights into the practice of how these contextures are being arranged within integrated-care partnerships. Three analysis steps achieve this: (1) the formulating interpretation, (2) the reflecting interpretation and (3) the constant comparative analysis (for details on method description, see Jansen and Poranzke, pp. 000–0 in this book).

Data collection and analyses

The data that has been analysed for this paper was conducted in qualitative, semi-structured interviews. Seventeen persons in hospitals of metropolitan areas in northern Germany (Hamburg, Bremen and Osnabrück) were interviewed. These persons are either case managers or social workers and work in the field of hospital discharge, i.e. their professional context is embedded into integrated-care partnerships and interface management. In case of a sequential analytical approach like the one suggested by the documentary method, computer-aided data analysis (i.e. software such as

MAXQDA) does not provide much benefits over a 'pen and paper' procedure.[6] Thus, the data analysis was carried out by directly working with the text documents.

Results

The following data analysis aims at describing the different contextures (market, hierarchy, health-care delivery, network and so on) and how the involved parties in integrated-care partnerships arrange these contextures.

Market and hierarchic demands in integrated-care partnerships

Hospitals in particular face strong market demands due to the DRG remuneration system. As an external demand, the length of hospitalisation becomes a superordinated factor that has major impacts on the hospital discharge planning. Patients have to be discharged in time if hospitals do not want financial penalties. This affects the cooperation with follow-up care institutions such as rehab centres, nursing homes and so on. Mr Smith, a case manager, gives following description of the DRG system and the related impacts on his work.[7]

> It [the DRG system] is great for the workflows. We do not plan workflows on a gut level nor just for medical reasons. We have to take into account the DRG remuneration when it comes to cooperation and integrated care, because the DRG system dictates an average hospitalisation for each patient. Complying with these limits is our duty because it's required by the health-care insurance companies. We have to respect this. Sometimes this situation is not what we want. And sometimes it's against the patients' wishes. And sometimes, quite rarely, it's also against our company's opinion.

The DRG system becomes a structural element that 'embeds' the integrated-care partnership into a timeframe wherein the cooperation and coordination tasks have to be accomplished. It is superordinated in the way that the timeframe appears as restricted element and 'duty'. This affects the involved actors in different ways. First of all, this mostly affects 'us', i.e. the 'network' persons or case managers, who are in contact with other companies in the context of integrated-care partnerships. Sometimes it affects patients, and quite rarely the company is affected. The DRG system leads to a 'disturbance sensitivity' in hospital discharge planning that sets the highest pressure on case managers. However, it is still considered as positive ('It is great for the workflows') because it can be used as a pressurising medium to control and optimise workflows. The DRG system is an immutable external directive that, at a first glance, limits the scope of actions but that at last offers new opportunities of professional autonomy and control.

> Anyway, reasonably shaping or structuring the workflows according to all concerns: patient wishes and orientation, clinical pathways, a constant high-level medical treatment of patients and the pinpoint of hospital discharge, all these are supported by a successful cooperation. Apart from that, a harmonic rapport has positive effects on the working atmosphere that leads to less workload. I can simply call and say, 'Hey pal, I have someone for you for admission, you already know him…' That's much easier than any bureaucratic procedures. And working like this simply makes more fun.

On the one hand, well-planned and precise workflows, which become a necessity due to the DRG system, have positive impacts on the collaboration of the team by establishing structures. On the other hand, uncomplicated and unconstrained ways of collaboration and cooperation are preferred. At first glance, this seems incompatible. However, the DRG system might function as a tool to realise professional autonomy. A fluent workflow without bureaucratic barriers seems to be more easily established in loosely coupled networks where each actor has enough capacity for decision-making. The DRG system serves as 'controlling frame' that ensures (voluntary) liability of network partners with no need for contractual bindings. Thus, there is enough leeway for the network partners to frame the network structures and make their own decisions.

Mr Smith, however, rejects contractual bindings, since they are connected with disadvantages.

> It's something completely different when a good, informal cooperation changes into tight contractual bindings or a little circle of wagons with only a limited amount of companies that seal themselves off from the others. Well, you may see advantages like an information highway for patients' data in such cases. But the disadvantages in contractual bound cooperation overweigh quite clearly.

This emphasises the importance of professional autonomy in integrated-care partnerships for the involved actors. Contractual cooperations are seen opposite to 'good, informal cooperation'. The disadvantages of exclusive cooperation networks are first related to market and competition and second to the scope of action, which should not be limited by too strong regulations.

> If a good cooperation leads to exclusivity, it has very negative impacts on the market and causes considerable perturbations amongst the competitors. It also narrows the scope of action we have. Cooperation is great and structuring workflows as well. But exclusive cooperations – only you and no one else – that's nothing, I don't like that. So, regarding this point I like to keep this boundary of my work untouched.

Integrated-care partnerships, where the involved actors do not pursue own interests at the expense of others, enable sustainable network structures.

> Sustainability in terms of partnership means that when there is a form of partnership with a common mission, the commonness of this mission is appreciated by all partners. The mission is to accompany the patient on his way and not to say: This is my provision of service and duty, and that is yours, good luck! We have to realise the binding component, the job of reasonably accompanying the patient – which is, in the end, of course our duty towards the health insurances, too. And if we work together to pursue the goals of these missions and realise that this work is under a permanent development process, we can establish sustainable networks. Sustainability has something to do with freedom of choice and autonomy in contrast to consortiums and exclusive networks. They may be sustainable as well, but not in the way I think of.

Professional autonomy seems to be a core aspect of sustainable network structures. Lose couplings in networks ensure flexibility and keep spheres of influence for the involved network partners but also lead to an increased quality of care and of service provision if the 'binding component' is realised by all parties. The structures of integrated-care partnerships develop further and become stable if the 'freedom of choice and autonomy' is kept. Sustainable networks emerge when certain degrees of flexibility lose couplings and mutual reliability is present.

Self-interests in integrated-care partnerships

The next case is Mrs Johnson, who gives an example of how self-interest in cooperation networks is pursued and how this affects the negotiations of uprising tasks. Mrs Johnson is a case manager in a hospital and describes the discharge planning for (medically) 'complicated patients'. In such a case, it is considered a necessity to get in personal contact with the cooperation partners in order to get an impression of their quality of work. This helps to avoid unpleasant surprises in the patient's care provision.

> Sometimes, we also discharge patients in a persistent vegetative state (PVS) into nursing homes. In such cases, I always request a personal visit. They have to come to us. And if they don't want to come to us and see the patient, they simply don't get him, quite easy! Especially with patients in a PVS it is important for nursing homes to see the patients and get an impression of their physical state. Otherwise, they probably say, 'Oh no, I didn't know that he's so ill and has such a complicated ailment!' We have already had such troubles in the past, and patients had to be rehospitalised because the nursing home did not know how to cope with such patients. And you never know to whom you are

talking to on the phone, whether it's care staff or just a trainee who has no idea about the diagnosis and its implication for the treatment. So, now, for each patient with at least care level 2, someone from the nursing home has to come to us and see the patient. And they have to talk with the patient about the costs that arise in the nursing home and about possibilities of financial support. And it's the nursing homes that have to support the patient with the filing of applications for financial benefits from the insurances or social-welfare offices. I mean, if they don't want to do this, they want the money from the patients, right? They have to make sure that the patients can pay the stay in the nursing home. And if they say it's not their task to file applications (well, after all, it is indeed not their task to do this), but if they don't take over this task, the patient will not move into their institution. You really have to look closely at your cooperation partners. And we have good cooperations with some nursing homes, where we can say, 'We have a new patient for you, no application for a care level made yet, but I can tell you the care insurance will grant payments for sure.' And in this way, we have good cooperations with several nursing homes and were able to perform discharge of patients at short notice into these nursing homes. And those who didn't want to do it this way are no longer our cooperation partners.

The description of the cooperation starts with an example of the discharge planning of severely dependent patients. The discharge planning of such patients is always risky because follow-up care institutions may not be prepared to provide adequate care for those patients. This may lead to so-called 'revolving door effects' (recommitments of patients) and financial disadvantages for the hospital.

This perspective comes from an *organisational* point of view, where additional tasks (personal visits of patients) are requested from the cooperation partners to avoid additional costs (recommitment) for the company. In the course of the conversation, Mrs Johnson's perspective changes from an organisational to a personal level. In case the cooperation partner is not willing to take over additional paperwork (filing of application), the patient will not be discharged into their institution. Unpopular tasks, which typically lie in the area of responsibility of Mrs Johnson, are moved over to the cooperation partners. She aims at negotiating common tasks to gain benefits in terms of personal favour.

To pursue her own interests, Mrs Johnson puts not only network partners under pressure but also health insurances. Concerning cost objectives, health insurances normally would be considered as most 'powerful' in the network structure and controlling the cooperation process by determining the financial framework. However, Mrs Johnson threatens insurances with increasing costs in case the health insurance will not react.

The department says, 'On 18th July the patient can be discharged, from a medical point of view.' Then I take a look at the documents and think, hey, it would be quite fine for us if we could discharge him a day earlier. I call the department and talk to the doctor: can we transfer him on 17 July? Yes? And then I cross out the 18 and replace it with 17, and that's the final discharge date. And then I ask the partners, 'Can we transfer the patient to you by then?' And they give feedback if they can take the patient or not, or why it's not possible, for example, it does not work because the patient's bed has not been provided yet, health insurance did not grant it. OK, then I call the health insurance and say, 'Well, we either lay your patient on the ground, which will not be very cheap for you because then he will have many new problems, or you grant the bed quite quickly and send the documents via fax so we can order the bed.' And this mostly works.

This example shows a very painstaking way of 'optimising' the date of patients' hospital discharges. The discharge is planned completely with regard to the length of hospitalisation. From the patients' point of view, the only concern seems to be whether it is medically reasonable. The patients are not included in the discharge-planning decision-making. All conversations in this context are either made with doctors ('Can we transfer him earlier?') or the network collaborators ('Can we transmit the patient to you by then?'). Furthermore, we can clearly see how pressure is exerted on network partners by negotiating *costs*. With respect to nursing homes, the consideration is that they need new 'customers', so they are willing to take over additional tasks. The joint basis of mutual trust and cooperation is continually given up in favour of personal benefits. Mrs Johnson cleverly manages pushing through her own interests when negotiating common network tasks.

Mutual expectations in integrated-care partnerships

The next example is an interview conducted with two persons at the same time, Mr Frank and Mrs Taylor. They both attach importance to mutual reliability and support in the context of hospital discharge planning. Based on experience, they try to find the appropriate service provider for the follow-up care of patients.

MRS TAYLOR: I really want to see the patient in good hands. And I think we have developed a good instinct which provider fits to a patient. For instance, we have partners that are very good in treating junkies. They really get along very well with them. However, this would not be the best provider for an old, anxious grandma. And this works really well, the concession to saying, we look after the administrative stuff and we expect from you that you'll take our patient. And this is clear for both sides.

The cooperation is based on respect and trust. Thus, mutual expectations are established and ensure an informal way of working together. The negotiation of tasks and cooperation is not bound to regulations or contracts. With regard to the network partners, Mrs Taylor talks about expectations ('we expect') and not about obligations. The expectations are 'clear for both sides', which means that over time mutual reliability has developed.

Mr Frank reports from local meetings for service providers where the development of care and supply structures as well as integrated-care partnerships is discussed. According to Mr Frank, these meetings help to build stable and sustainable network structures.

MR FRANK: We have working groups with different topics, with a certain circle of people who regularly meet. And this really is sustainable cooperation. Because due to this cooperation we see and know each other, we can informally discuss problems with no need for bureaucratic procedures. This really fosters stable cooperations.

In integrated-care partnerships, as described by Mr Frank, informal negotiations are preferred over contractual obligations. On the one hand, this ensures that professional autonomy of all involved actors is kept. On the other hand, the mutual reliability eases the cooperation. To conclude, we can say that sustainable integrated-care partnerships rely on expectations and reliability, are less regulated and allow network structures to be flexible. By fathoming out mutual expectations, these structures become stable.

Integrated-care partnerships do not need contractual regulations; they are 'self-regulating' – or self-organising, to speak in systems-theoretical language. The mechanism for regulation works on a 'give-and-take basis'.

MR FRANK: On the one hand, we can realise short-term discharge of patients. And on the other hand, I think, well, they get new customers from us and thus, the other providers have financial benefits from these patients. I think, this can be considered as mutual give-and-take.

The cooperation is described as mutual give-and-take. This indicates a balanced power relationship between the partners. However, it seems that there is a more urgent necessity for the follow-up service providers to cooperate and a higher dependency from hospitals than vice versa. Hospitals can discharge patients at short notice, which seems to be a fine benefit. However, they are not restricted to a single cooperation partner. The follow-up service providers, meanwhile, face the economic necessity to get new customers only from hospitals.

MR FRANK: Well, we do not depend on the follow-up service providers in order to get new patients, not at all. Rather, our cooperation partners or the many nursing homes, they want our patients! And every now and

then they give us a call to say, hi there, we're still here and we offer this
and we have these services.

MRS TAYLOR: Yes, like, we haven't received any patients from you for so
long, how does it look like right now?

MR FRANK: Or they call to tell us how many free beds they have, and
so on.

MRS TAYLOR: And we say, nice to hear from you, we'll inform our colleagues about this.

We can see a clear statement that points out the advantageous initial position of hospitals in the context of integrated-care partnerships and discharge planning. This could be used by hospitals to their advantage to push
through their own interests. Mrs Taylor and Mr Frank do not abuse their
advantage in order to push tasks over to network partners. However, they
try to control the network in order to change the mutual expectations with
regard to patient-centred care. As briefly mentioned in the first citation (and
more emphasised in other paragraphs of the interview that have not been
cited here), they prefer providers that fulfil the patients' needs, and thus they
expect a certain degree of patient orientation from their network partners.
This shows that, beyond hierarchical or market demands, networks appear
as their own mechanism to control integrated-care partnerships, ensuring
the self-organisation of such systems.

Discussion

We have said that cooperation becomes increasingly important to ensure a
comprehensive supply of (chronically) ill people because the structure of the
health-care sector is heavily fragmented. With respect to a sustainable interface management, the question is which factors influence the negotiations
of tasks within a cooperation network. In integrated-care partnerships, each
party is exposed to polycontextural conditions in such a way that the concurrent presence of hierarchic, bureaucratic determination, economic and
medical requirements has to be incorporated into the network structures
to stabilise the network. The DRG system as economic contexture represents a strong outside disturbance for hospitals, because its impact can be
located both on a hierarchical and a market level. In the first case, it is
the hospital's financial department that puts pressure on all other departments to discharge patients within a given time. In the latter case, since the
DRG system limits the average time of hospitalisation, hospitals no longer
benefit from patients' long stays but instead have to compete with other
hospitals and service providers in order to get as many patients as possible.
Then again, competition might enforce the establishment of cooperation
networks. Although DRGs apply only to hospitals, they have an impact
on the whole network and cooperation process. On the one hand, hospitals are interested in a well-planned discharge of patients to avoid financial

disadvantages due to the DRG system; on the other hand, other providers such as nursing homes or ambulatory services are interested in supporting hospitals with the transition of patients. This ensures the development of a good partnership and network, which also stands for new 'customers' from the hospitals in the future.

As we can see from the empirical data, networks appear as their own mechanism to control integrated-care partnerships beyond market aspects and bureaucratic determination. The actors in networks manage these contextures differently. For instance, one possible way to rearrange those contextures is to use the economic pressure built up by the DRG system to strengthen one's own position in a network. Mrs Johnson's example shows how she exercises control in favour of personal benefits. Another possibility could be a parasitical behaviour that 'abuses' the DRG system in order to control the network without appearing as ruler (see Mr Smith). The DRG system frames the workflows but does not narrow the scope of action. Rather, it opens possibilities for informal cooperation as long as network partner acts within the 'legal framework' created by the DRG system. In such an environment, network structures with loosely coupled elements can emerge.

Replacing 'lose couplings' in networks (reflexive contracts) with inflexible structures (contractual bindings) may lead to disadvantages in integrated care. Problems in health-care delivery may even be concealed by formal rules. Contractual bindings in networks that suppress the competitive environment may have negative consequences for patient-centred care.[8] A recent example for negative consequences of contractual bindings in cooperation relationships is the affair of the Helios hospitals in Berlin (BZ/dapd 2011; Bach and Radke 2011). The idea of network as control mechanism was dismissed and replaced by a 'network' consortium where the process of integrated care was planned and regulated in the context of hierarchical structures. In this case, the competition was influenced by inflexible network structures that included just a few actors and excluded many others. This affected the quality of patient provision because missing reflexive awareness and self-regulation of the network could not eliminate this drawback. Not least, regulated cooperation relationships mostly have a negative impact on the patients' autonomy of decisions (Dahm 2008). The more hospitals compete among each other, the more they depend on other providers (GPs, nursing homes, etc.) and their admissions of patients to hospitals or at least their recommendations for a certain hospital. When network partners have to take over tasks that usually belong to others at their own expense, they might choose to cooperate with other organisations in the future instead (competition) (Debatin and Puttfarcken 2008).

Sustainability in this context appears as reflection strategy for organisations to learn how to best combine two conflictive aims: first, gaining as much profit within a treatment network where many organisations are involved. Second, when negotiating necessary tasks with other network partners, doing this in such a way that one stays part of the network in the future. Professional autonomy in the context of reliability leads to integrated-care partnerships where 'the parties to a network agree to forego [sic] the right to pursue own interests at the expense of others' (Powell 2011: 35) and may lead to a better quality of care and patient provision.

Conclusions

The core question of this chapter was how dynamic structures of self-organisation in integrated-care partnerships can emerge via networks as mechanisms of mutual control and how these structures ensure a sustainable, comprehensive quality of health-care delivery. Networks, as 'reflexive contracts', promote sustainability in integrated-care partnerships by balancing the polycontextural conditions of medical and economic contextures under increasing pressure of the DRGs. The way in which the interviewed professional actors understand sustainability and put it into practice can be described as interplay of identity and control (White 2008). They enforce their claims towards not only other cooperation partners in the network but also themselves. They negotiate the different tasks that arise in the context of hospital discharge planning with their cooperation partners. They fathom advantages and disadvantages during the negotiations and appraise the cooperation partners' reactions in order to adjust their own decisions and actions.

Most notably, all questioned actors have similar ideas of how cooperation networks should be established. They point out the *informal character* of the relationship of network partners and the arrangement of network structures. All of them are against consortiums and do not think much of contractual relations. In their opinion, a network consists of 'loosely coupled' elements. A too-strong regimentation of cooperations restricts their formal arrangement and leeway in decision-making, which is contrary to the professional self-conception of the interviewed actors of how cooperation networks should work. Profit-seeking consortiums do not have the necessary reflexive awareness and adaptability. This may lead to an imbalance of the arrangement of medical and economic contextures in disfavour of the patient-centredness because inappropriate conditions and poor supply cannot be eliminated by self-regulation. Professional autonomy, however, is the basis for sustainable network structures and keeps these structures stable.[9] Autonomy enables informal levels of decision-finding, negotiations and agreements that allow flexible acting as circumstances demand. Network partners develop social structures of mutual trust and reliability, which then again permanently rebuilds the stability of an otherwise fragile network structure. Sustainability in networks, to summarise, can be described as autonomy (from the systems perspective) in the context of reliability (from the networks or environmental perspective).

Sustainability in networks, this is our conclusion, can especially be established by loose couplings (informal cooperation relationship) of network elements (cooperation partners). Thus, the conceded autonomy gives various options to the professional actors regarding their decision-making. When two cooperation partners cannot find a common basis for their relationship, other network partners will be chosen. This gives cause to all participating organisations to behave 'cooperatively' and keep their chance to further play an important role in a network of patient-centred care and healthcare provision.[10] The interviewed professionals called this a 'give-and-take basis' for their relationship towards other organisations. Sustainability and its practical implication by the professional actors might be considered as reflection strategy according to the stability and durability of integrated-care networks, also taking into account the point of 'staying in a network'.

Notes

1 Regarding the scientific system, for example, only truth (as single contexture) is relevant for scientific operations. Untruth just helps to reflect what appears as true and false. Judging what is true is not done by payments (economic system), governance (political system) or beliefs (religious system) but only with reference to scientific programmes such as methods and theories (Luhmann 1998).
2 'An organisation is polyphonic when it is connected to several function systems without a predefined primary function system' (Åkerstrøm Andersen 2003: 167).
3 The general systems theory by Bertalanffy (1976) considers systems as open; thus, the dynamics of systems are based on an exchange between systems and their environment. The relationship between system and environment is considered as an input–output scheme, with structures defining the roles of the transformation of this exchange. In contrast to Bertalanffy's approach, Luhmann does not consider systems as 'open'. Rather, he adopted concepts of self-organisation and later self-reference of systems (Foerster and Zopf 1962, Foerster 1976), which means that systems are operationally closed. A system has always to be observed in relation to its environment, which means the emergence of structures always depends on irritations from the environment (*order from noise*; see Foerster 1993).
4 The autopoiesis concept was invented by the biologist Maturana together with Varela, who explained how a cell can reproduce itself without direct input from its environment, since the cell itself is separated from the environment via its membranes (Maturana and Varela 1980, Maturana 1985). Luhmann applied the concept of autopoiesis and operational closure on social systems, which reproduce themselves by the basal operation of communication.
5 While Talcott Parsons' understanding of systems (1951) was very closely connected to *action*, Luhmann sees *communication* as the basic operation of systems. The key difference between action and communication as basal operations affects assumptions on causality. Considering action, it seems easier to identify motives as causes for these actions that correlate with certain effects (Lindemann 2006). Communication, by contrast, does not determine the social systems but keeps up a state of uncertainty where the ascertainment is achieved during the process of communication, which, again, creates new alternatives on how to proceed and thereby maintains the uncertainty (Baecker 2005). Effects in social systems cannot be explicitly assigned to specific causes (e.g., the motives of underlying actions).

6 Referencing in mailing list archive, available online at https://lists.fu-berlin.de/htdig/qsf_l/2010-October/msg00000.html.
7 Names have been changed to maintain anonymity. However, personal names are used for a better readability.
8 Competition can also be understood as quality indicator. Contractual bindings in networks means that other cooperation partners do not appear in the competitive environment any longer and have no chance to shape the networks structures by own claims and demands (identity and control).
9 This, by the way, goes along with the conception of operational closure of organisations.
10 That means each party in the network has to stick to the reflexive contract and 'use' the network to arrange the conflicting requirements of high quality in health care supply under the circumstances of limited (financial) resources.

References

Åkerstrøm Andersen, N. (2003) 'Polyphonic Organisations', in T. Bakken and T. Hernes (eds.), *Autopoietic Organization Theory: Drawing on Niklas Luhmann's Social Systems Perspective*, Oslo, Malmö and Herndon, Virg.: Abstrakt forlag, Liber Ekonomi and Copenhagen Business School Press, pp. 151–82.
——(2008) *Partnerships: Machines of Possibility*, Bristol: Policy Press.
BZ/dapd (2011) 'Helios-Klinik: Betrug? Razzia bei Helios-Klinik', *BZ-online*, 21 June.
Bach, I. and J. Radke (2011) 'Verdächtige Helios-Ärzte weiter im Dienst', *Der Tagesspiegel Online*, 24 June.
Baecker, D. (1997) 'Interfaces: A View from Social Systems Theory', paper presented at the Journée d'étude avec Harrison C. White, 'Social Embeddedness of Economic Transactions', Paris: Fondation Maison des Sciences de l'Homme.
——(2001) 'Kapital als strukturelle Kopplung', *Soziale Systeme*, 7 (2): 314–27.
——(2002) *Wozu Systeme?* Berlin: Kadmos.
——(2005) *Form und Formen der Kommunikation*, Frankfurt: Suhrkamp.
Bertalanffy, L. V. (1976) *General System Theory: Foundations, Development, Applications Foundations, Development, Applications*, rev. edn, New York: George Braziller Inc.
Besl, S. (2011) 'Moderne, vernetzte Versorgungsformen', in H. Kunhardt (ed.), *Systemisches Management im Gesundheitswesen*, Wiesbaden: Gabler, pp. 205–20.
Bohnsack, R. (2007) *Rekonstruktive Sozialforschung: Einführung in qualitative Methoden*, 8., durchges. Aufl. UTB, Stuttgart: Barbara Budrich.
——(2010)'Dokumentarische Methode und Typenbildung: Bezüge zur Systemtheorie', in R. John, A. Henkel, and J. Rückert-John (eds.), *Die Methodologien des Systems: Wie kommt man zum Fall und wie dahinter?* Wiesbaden: VS-Verlag für Sozialwissenschaften, pp. 291–320.
Bräutigam, C., N. Klettke, W. Kunstmann, A. Prietz and M. Sieger (2005) 'Versorgungskontinuität durch Pflegeüberleitung? Ergebnisse einer teilnehmenden Beobachtung', *Pflege*, 18 (2): 112–20.
Brunsson, N. (1985) *The Irrational Organization: Irrationality as a Basis for Organizational Action and Change*, Chicester: John Wiley & Sons Ltd.
Brunsson, N., A. Rasche and D. Seidl (2012) 'The Dynamics of Standardization: Three Perspectives on Standards in Organization Studies', *Organization Studies*, 33 (5–): 613–32.

Bühler, E. (2006) 'Kooperation fit für die Zukunft', in E. Bühler (ed.), *Überleitungsmanagement und Integrierte Versorgung: Brücke zwischen Krankenhaus und nachstationärer Versorgung*, Stuttgart: Kohlhammer, pp. 11–28.

Dahm, F.-J. (2008) 'Unzulässiger Kooperationsvertrag zwischen Krankenhaus und Arzt', *Der Urologe A*, 47 (10): 1353–6.

Debatin, J. F. and M. Puttfarcken (2008) 'Gute Medizin auch unter wachsendem Wettbewerbsdruck', in N. Klusen and A. Meusch (eds.), *Zukunft der Krankenhausversorgung: Qualität, Wettbewerb und neue Steuerungsansätze im DRG-Systen*, Baden-Baden: Nomos, pp. 225–35.

Drucker, P. (2001) 'Next Society', *Economist*, 1 November.

Dt. Caritasverband (ed.) (2005) *Versorgungskontinuität durch Entlassungsmanagement: Empfehlungen zur sektorenübergreifenden Vernetzung von Krankenhäusern, ambulanten Pflegediensten und weiteren nachsorgenden Einrichtungen*. Dt. Caritasverband.

Foerster, H. von (1976) 'Objects: Tokens for (Eigen-)Behaviors', *ASC Cybernetics Forum*, 8 (3 and 4): 91–6.

——(1993) *Wissen und Gewissen: Versuch einer Brücke*, Frankfurt: Suhrkamp.

Foerster, H. V. and G. W. Zopf (1962) *Principles of Self-Organization: Transactions*, Oxford: Symposium Publications, Pergamon Press.

Freidson, E. (1980) *Doctoring Together: A Study of Professional Social Control*, Chicago, Ill.: University of Chicago Press.

——(2007) *Professional Dominance: The Social Structure of Medical Care*, New Brunswick, NJ: Aldine Transaction.

Fuchs, P. (2008a) 'Prävention: Zur Mythologie und Realität einer paradoxen Zuvorkommenheit', in I. Saake and W. Vogd (eds.), *Moderne Mythen der Medizin: Studien zur organisierten Krankenhausbehandlung*, Wiesbaden: VS-Verlag für Sozialwissenschaften, pp. 363–78.

——(2008b) 'Nachhaltige Entwicklung: theoretisch', available online at www.fen. ch/texte/gast_fuchs_nachhaltigkeit.pdf (accessed 21 July 2014).

Glaeske, G. (2002) 'Integrierte Versorgung in Deutschland: Rahmenbedingungen für mehr Effektivität und Effizienz?' in K.-J. Preuß, J. Räbiger, J. Sommer, and H. Andersen (eds.), *Managed Care: Evaluation und Performance-Measurement integrierter Versorgunsmodelle – Stand der Entwicklung in der EU, der Schweiz und den USA*, Stuttgart: Schattauer, pp. 3–19.

Glasby, G. P. (2002) 'Sustainable Development: The Need for a New Paradigm', *Environment, Development and Sustainability*, 4 (4): 333–45.

Grossmann, R. and K. Scala (eds.) (2002a) *Intelligentes Krankenhaus: Innovative Beispiele der Organisationsentwicklung in Krankenhäusern und Pflegeheimen*, New York and Vienna: Springer.

——(2002b) 'Krankenhäuser als Organisationen steuern und entwickeln', in R. Grossmann and K. Scala (eds.), *Intelligentes Krankenhaus: Innovative Beispiele der Organisationsentwicklung in Krankenhäusern und Pflegeheimen*, New York and Vienna: Springer, pp. 12–31.

Günther, G. (1979) 'Life as Polycontexturality', in G. Günther (ed.), *Beiträge zur Grundlegung einer operationsfähigen Dialektik*, Hamburg: Meiner, pp. 283–306.

Hafferty, F. W. and D. W. Light (1995) 'Professional Dynamics and the Changing Nature of Medical Work', *Journal of Health and Social Behavior*, special issue, pp. 132–53.

Heaton, J., A. Corden and G. Parker (2012) '"Continuity of Care": A Critical Interpretive Synthesis of How the Concept Was Elaborated by a National Research Programme', *International Journal of Integrated Care*, 12: 1–9.

Herwartz, H. and C. Strumann (2013) 'Hospital Efficiency under Prospective Reimbursement Schemes: An Empirical Assessment for the Case of Germany', *The European Journal of Health Economics: HEPAC: Health Economics in Prevention and Care*, 15 (2): 175–86.

Jansen, T. and W. Vogd (2013) 'Polykontexturale Verhältnisse: disjunkte Rationalitäten am Beispiel von Organisationen', *Zeitschrift für Theoretische Soziologie*, 1: 82–97.

Kaehr, R. (1993) 'Disseminatorik: Zur Logik der "Second Order Cybernetics": Von den "Laws of Form" zur Logik der Reflexionsform', in D. Baecker (ed.), *Kalkül der Form*, Frankfurt: Suhrkamp, pp. 152–96.

Kölking, H. (2007) 'Entwicklung der Gesundheitswirtschaft in Deutschland', in H. Kölking (ed.), *DRG und Strukturwandel in der Gesundheitswirtschaft*, Stuttgart: Kohlhammer, pp. 19–31.

Kurlemann, U. (2010) 'Entlassungsmanagement', *Der Gynäkologe*, 43 (10): 832–8.

Laloe, F. (2007) 'Modelling Sustainability: From Applied to Involved Modeling', *Social Science Information*, 46 (1): 87–107.

Lindemann, G. (2006) 'Handlung, Interaktion, Kommunikation', in A. Scherr (ed.), *Soziologische Basics: Eine Einführung für Pädagogen und Pädagoginnen*, Wiesbaden: VS-Verlag für Sozialwissenschaften, pp. 67–73.

Luhmann, N. (1984) *Soziale Systeme: Grundriß einer allgemeinen Theorie*, Frankfurt: Suhrkamp.

——(1992) 'Operational Closure and Structural Coupling: The Differentiation of the Legal System', *Cardozo Law Review*, 13 (5): 1419–41.

——(1994) *Die Wirtschaft der Gesellschaft*, 6th edn, Frankfurt: Suhrkamp.

——(1996) *Social Systems*, Palo Alto, Calif.: Stanford University Press.

——(1998) *Die Wissenschaft der Gesellschaft*, 3rd edn, Frankfurt: Suhrkamp.

——(2000) *Organisation und Entscheidung*, Opladen: Westdeutscher Verlag.

——(2005) 'Der medizinische Code', *Soziologische Aufklärung 5: Konstruktivistische Perspektiven*, Wiesbaden: VS-Verlag für Sozialwissenschaften, pp. 176–88.

Luks, F. (2002) *Nachhaltigkeit*, Hamburg: Europäische Verlagsanstalt.

March, J. G. and J. P. Olsen (1979) *Ambiguity and Choice in Organizations*, 2nd edn, Bergen: Universitetsforlaget.

Maturana, H. R. (1985) *Erkennen: Die Organisation und Verkörperung von Wirklichkeit*, 2nd edn, Braunschweig and Wiesbaden: Vieweg.

Maturana, H. R. and F. Varela (1980) *Autopoiesis and Cognition: The Realization of the Living*, Boston, Mass.: Springer Netherlands.

McKinlay, J. B. (1977) 'The Business of Good Doctoring or Doctoring as Good Business: Reflections on Freidson's View of the Medical Game', *International Journal of Health Services: Planning, Administration, Evaluation*, 7 (3): 459–88.

Ommen, O., B. Ullrich, C. Janßen and H. Pfaff (2007) 'Die ambulant-stationäre Schnittstelle in der medizinischen Versorgung', *Medizinische Klinik: Intensivmedizin und Notfallmedizin*, 102 (11): 913–17.

Parsons, T. (1951) *The Social System*, New York: Free Press.

Powell, W. W. (2011) 'Neither Market Nor Hierarchy: Network Forms of Organization', in M. Godwyn and J. H. Gittell (eds.), *Sociology of Organizations: Structures and Relationships*, Thousand Oaks, Calif.: Pine Forge Press, pp. 30–40.

Quentin, W., D. Scheller-Kreinsen, M. Blümel, A. Geissler and R. Busse (2013) 'Hospital Payment Based on Diagnosis-Related Groups Differs in Europe and Holds Lessons for the United States', *Health Affairs (Project Hope)*, 32 (4): 713–23.

Sadler, W. A. (2001) *Fliegend in die Fünfziger*, Düsseldorf and Zürich: Walter-Verlag.

Schaeffer, D. and M. Ewers (2006) 'Integrierte Versorgung nach deutschem Muster', *Pflege and Gesellschaft*, 11 (3): 197–209.

Simon, F. B. (2007) *Einführung in die systemische Organisationstheorie*, Heidelberg: Carl-Auer-Verlag.

Stock, S., E. Plamper, M. Redaèli, A. Gerber and K. W. Lauterbach (2005) 'Versorgungspolitische Ziele der Integrierten Versorgung', in J. Klauber, B.-P. Robra and H. Schnellschmidt (eds.), *Wege aus der Krise der Versorgungssituation: Beiträge aus der Versorgungsforschung*, Bern: Huber, pp. 85–98.

Vogd, W. (2008) 'Paradoxien einer chirurgischen Abteilung: Wenn leitende Akteure zugleich entscheiden und funktionieren sollen', in I. Saake and W. Vogd (eds.), *Moderne Mythen der Medizin: Studien zur organisierten Krankenhausbehandlung* (Wiesbaden: VS-Verlag für Sozialwissenschaften), pp. 109–36.

——(2009a) 'Braucht die neue Medizin das Subjekt? Überlegungen zur Organisation der Krankenbehandlung im Zeitalter des New Public Management', in K. Mozygemba, S. Mümken, U. Krause, M. Zündel, M. Rehm, N. Höfling-Engels, D. Lüdecke and B. Qurban (eds.), *Nutzerorientierung: Ein Fremdwort in der Gesundheitssicherung?* Bern: Huber, pp. 113–20.

——(2009b) *Rekonstruktive Organisationsforschung: Qualitative Methodologie und theoretische Integration – eine Einführung*, Opladen: Verlag Barbara Budrich.

——(2009c) 'Systemtheorie und Methode? Zum komplexen Verhältnis von Theoriearbeit und Empirie in der Organisationsforschung', *Soziale Systeme*, 15 (1): 97–136.

——(2010) 'Methodologie und Verfahrensweise der dokumentarischen Methode und ihre Kompatibilität zur Systemtheorie', in R. John, A. Henkel, and J. Rückert-John (eds.), *Die Methodologien des Systems: Wie kommt man zum Fall und wie dahinter?* Wiesbaden: VS-Verlag für Sozialwissenschaften, pp. 121–40.

——(2012) 'Versorgungsstrukturen und Patientenrolle im Wandel der Medizin und des Gesundheitssystems', *Monitor Versorgungsforschung*, 5 (4): 38–40.

Weick, K. E. (1995) *Sensemaking in Organizations*, Thousand Oaks, Calif.: Sage.

Weick, K. E., K. M. Sutcliffe and D. Obstfeld (2005) 'Organizing and the Process of Sensemaking', *Organization Science*, 16 (4), 409–21.

Wetzel, R. (2005) 'Hintergründe und Steuerungspotenziale der Nachhaltigkeit. Ein systemtheoretischer Blick', in K. Großmann, U. Hahn and J. Schröder (eds.), *Im Prinzip Nachhaltigkeit. Akteurskonstellationen und Handlungsspielräume in interdisziplinärer Betrachtung*, Munich: Rainer Hampp Verlag, pp. 189–210.

White, H. C. (2008) *Identity and Control: How Social Formations Emerge*, 2nd edn, Princeton, NJ: Princeton University Press.

Wingenfeld, K. (2002) 'Der Übergang des Krankenhauspatienten in die ambulante Pflege', in D. Schaeffer and M. Ewers (eds.), *Ambulant vor stationär: Perspektiven für eine integrierte ambulante Pflege Schwerstkranker*, Bern, Göttingen, Seattle and Toronto: Verlag Hans Huber, pp. 336–64.

Part IV
Reflections

8 The multiplication and realisation of speakers as polyphony

Armin Nassehi, Irmhild Saake and Katharina Mayr

Health-care ethics committees (HECs) are bodies within hospitals in which the practice of hospitals becomes observed in terms of ethics and moral distinctions. But maybe their ethical self-description is only half the truth, because their practice surpasses ethical functions in the narrow sense of the word. HECs can be characterised as the reaction of medical organisations to the demands of society to interrupt the professional decision-making by medical experts by asking questions which do not occur when cases only become observed by the professional means experts have available for their practice. We can observe something similar in businesses, where the communication of values and missions have come into vogue, or in scientific practice, where research programmes have to be accredited not only by scientific means but also concerning the ethical implications of the research. All these observations of medical or business or research practices use other means and logics than their own categories. At first glance this can be described as a case of *polyphonic organisations*, as Niels Åkerstrøm Andersen (2001) puts it. He says 'that many of society's systems such as art, politics, and education, have exploded beyond their organisational boundaries, and in effect a large number of new organisations have become aestheticised, politicised, and educationalised' (Åkerstrøm Andersen 2001: 3). This statement suggests that organisations formerly were social systems characterised by only one function, so, for example, business companies were organisations with only economical operations, universities with only scientific operations, or hospitals with only medical ones. We agree with Åkerstrøm Andersen that a wider mutual interference of function systems can be observed. And we also agree with his diagnosis that the logics and conditions of other function systems begin to penetrate and to infiltrate the practice of function systems. But as only a little deviation from this argument, we suggest that it is more the self-description of organisations that has changed into a more pluralistic form than the basic operations of function systems. Doubtlessly, the moral and political demands of society begin to have a stronger impact on organisations. And it is also true that, for example, businesses become observed as political actors – and doubtlessly they are. What has changed is the way in which organisations are able to describe themselves. Maybe it was possible for a business to reject all political demands by referring on its shape as a company, this is not possible any more. But it is not applicable to assert that organisations in classical modernity were monofunctional organisations. On the contrary, we argue that the societal function of organisations is to bring different functional logics of society together, not to harmonise them but to come to terms with the different practices of modern societies. So, for example, a hospital is by no means a medical organisation. Besides its medical categories, it also comprises economical, legal, scientific, religious and other operations. From a systems-theoretical point of view, this does not mean that organisations are able to de-differentiate the functional differentiation of society. On the contrary, organisations are the sites where functional differentiation becomes operated practically. Organisations are the sites where the different demands of the different functional logics clash – sometimes violently, sometimes nearly invisibly, sometimes harmonically, but always inevitably, as differences. To speak of *polyphony* as Åkerstrøm Andersen puts it might bear more truth than the notions explicitly wanted to express. Of course, organisations always have been polyoperative or polycontextural social systems, but now they are also polyphone (the Greek *phonē* refers to voice or sound). Polyphonic organisations in that sense are organisations in which it is no longer possible to enforce monocontextural self-descriptions. What we can hear from and within organisations is a polyphony of descriptions that thwarts former traditions of self-descriptions.

The example of hospital might be very characteristic for this. Especially the self-descriptions in the language of physicians with their professional ability to concentrate all the different aspects of hospital practices in the ethos of physicians and of medical expertise comes under fire. HECs are examples of how an organisation deals with new demands of descriptions, with new speaker positions and with the problem of how to come to terms with different voices.

In the following we want to analyse these different speaker positions. But before we can do that we have to reflect on the question, on what is meant by ethics. Although the practice of HECs surpasses ethical practices in the narrow sense of the word, it is necessary to refer to a sociological view on ethics, because the idea of HECs, the achievement of their foundations and, not least, the communicated motifs of actors in hospitals to be engaged in HECs or to bring them into being mostly have an ethical semantical shape. Thus, it is worthwhile to look at the semantic sources of these motifs and of the conditions of connectivity of ethical communication offers.

A commonplace assumption

Before starting research in the field of ethics, a few common assumptions need to be cleared up. The first is so common that it needs very little space at all: *ethics is an academic discipline*. This accurately describes its location and the problems it covers in a modern, functionally differentiated society.

As a branch of philosophy and a normative science, its frame of reference is initially located in a world of possible competing reasons. The basic problem is trying to explain good reasons – and the horizon is the sayability of ethical sentences which, even when they reflect an ethical practice, open up a *scientific* horizon. Ethics is therefore a science, and, like every science, it can only solve scientific problems (Luhmann 2002: 79–93). Practical problems are also the scientific problems of ethics, and that is not a deficiency but rather a consequence of the basic structure of modern society. A modern society cut loose from political, economic, legal, scientific, artistic, educational and medical problems on the one hand allows these disconnected spheres to relate radically to each other while on the other hand making them logically incompatible. This can be regarded as the fundamental character of societal modernity (Luhmann 1998: 1–21; Nassehi 2005a). This should first be understood before venturing into research on ethics.

An integrating function cannot be attributed to morals for the simple reason that most forms of order in modern society do not appear immoral but rather *amoral*. On the other hand, this is exactly the prerequisite for philosophical-ethical attempts at providing universal and collectively acceptable ethical figures with reasons, which, in turn, can achieve a rational status open, for instance, to criticism (Nassehi 2001). Modern ethical reflection, irrespective of its theoretical form, with its posit of acceptability, or at least of procedural implementation in political processes of operative coordination, can be seen as a reaction to the very pluralism of world views, ways of life and basic intuitions of the 'good life', which first produced the conditions for the disintegration of morality's clear claim to validity. The interdisciplinary form of ethical debates then is an expression of this diversification of ethical argumentation. They range from the philosophical reflection of the rationality of ethical judgements to figures of reasoning from applied ethics. They specialise not only in demonstrating their 'practical' efficacy but also in theological reflections on the significance of the religious content of 'unconditional' figures of rationality under conditions of differentiated modernity. The juridical and legal theoretical assertion of the accountability of legal entities (bodies, persons) creates subjects of moral judgement. In other words, the reflective form of an ethical practice of rationality based on good reasons reacts in the final instance to the fact that hardly any undisputed good reasons can be found for these or for maxims of action found in societal practice – in as far as this holds true, the reason must be separated into an ethical form of reflection which in turn takes on a scientific form.

Our argument uses the standard distinction between ethics and morals from the field of philosophical ethics: *ethics* as a form of a *morality*, which in turn need not be conscious of itself but simply applies empirically (or not as the case may be). It should be abundantly clear that this is a heuristic distinction. It is only used to determine the different worlds we are talking about here: *on the one hand* the moral world, in which a certain form of morality applies and which has to arm itself with rigor to gain validity;

on the other hand the reasoning world of ethics which does not perpetuate itself though the enforcement of moral standards but rather through its argumentative reasoning or ability to reason. Here we follow Niklas Luhmann's characterisation of morality as a form of communication that avails itself of the respect or disrespect towards individuals, in order to qualify their behaviour as good or bad (Luhmann 1996). So it is not a question of morality as a certain substance or quality but solely a question of moral communication in the sociological sense, i.e. it is a question of forms of communication that command moral respect or disrespect. The following point is decisive here: it is not that one is an empirical world while the other provides its reflections; rather we are dealing here with two empirical cases, with the moral regulation of actions and speaking as well as the practical business of reasoning.

Practical consequences

The interdisciplinarity and differentiation of ethical reflection in theoretical and practical research concurrently reflects the *practical conditions of ethical decision-making*. Similar to the way in which the practice of academic ethics hinted at here can be determined in social terms, it is of particular relevance for ethics research to demonstrate *the empirical conditions and locations* under which and by which ethical decisions are made in modern society. Such a research perspective does not negate the possibilities and necessity to search for good reasons. But it assumes that, to paraphrase Wittgenstein, no practical ethical problem can be solved even with the final explication of the best reasons, except the practical problem of philosophical reasoning. As said before, this is not an argument against the explication of reasons, which is a very specific type of practice and not an external observation. It is, rather, a plea for a supplementary and truly sociological, i.e. *empirical research* perspective. We are definitely *not* dealing here with the question of the rationality of good reasons; nor is it a question of the application of general ethical theoretical forms to concrete fields of 'applied ethics'; in other words, we are not talking about implementation questions but rather about the *societal conditions under which ethical decisions can be* practically *made in modern society*.

The subject of this paper is not *which* good reasons or philosophically reasonable maxims or virtues we can use to deal with certain problems but rather *how* ethical arguing and decision-making work in practice, how the appropriate forms of practice become established and under which conditions, in which concrete locations, which forms of ethical reflection prove to be empirically plausible and who becomes established as a legitimate speaker, as well as where and how. This question includes the query how communicative offers and arguments become observed as ethical statements because this is the source of 'ethical' motifs, attributions and claims. And when we locate the sites of ethical decision-making in modern society we come upon organisations, which face their polyphonic conditions of self-description.

The location of the ethical decision

The place in which ethical decisions which have consequences for practice are made in Western-type societies is not only the location of moral intuitions of a private way of life nor is it the ethos of professionals. Rather, more than anywhere else, it is in the area of biomedical and biotechnical research and practice, by no means owing allegiance only to the new biotechnical opportunities but also to the pluralism of ethical perspectives and the loss of the ethical justification of the classical professional role, especially in the medical sphere.

The empirical location of such ethical decisions is usually the ethical committee, in other words institutionally supported bodies. Here, under organisational conditions, a particular style of ethical reflection has become established in the shape of the following committees: in clinical ethics committees and commissions, in the ethics committees of professional associations, in the ethics committees of scientific associations, in commissions of enquiry in parliamentary decision-making processes, in public discourses, especially on bioethical issues, in ethic committees at the federal state level and even in large companies. What all these forms of practice have in common is that they do not do exactly what would be expected of fervent moralists with fundamentalist interests. It can be observed empirically that in such communication contexts it is the limits of the final moral claim that become clear in the face of decision-oriented, i.e. practice-relevant ethical forms of reflection (van den Daele 2001a, 2001b).

It is particularly interesting that in these forms of practice ethical decisions by no means copy the routines and patterns of arguments of scientific and academic reflection on ethical questions. Nor do they involve anything like a theory–practice transfer. Instead, a unique form of communication has become established which of itself has taken on a kind of ethical quality. This can be witnessed, for instance, in public hearings of the national ethics committee or in the proceedings of HECs.

The typical participants in such committees are not exclusively ethics experts. Despite the growing need for ethical expertise and the development of decision-making processes, there did not occur an operative demarcation between ethicists and other professions. Rather, the ethical decision-making process has become a genuine *interdisciplinary* process, in the sense not of different academic disciplines but of different professional groups. Their *practical interdisciplinarity* does not just decide and reflect *on* the ethical debate and its reasonable arguments, its interdisciplinary form of communication and its differentiated memberships *is its ethical practice itself – beyond ethical reasoning in terms of academic practices.*

The aim of the research perspective being followed here is, therefore, to research the empirical implementation conditions of ethical decisions supported by committees and to gain an insight into the social, organisational structure of the forms of decisions rather than of the ethical decision-making algorithms and levels of reasoning. Beyond that there are also various political and legal conditions of ethical boards, such as HECs, but also other bodies on regional, national and transnational levels. This paper does not focus on these conditions but on the organisational conditions of the social processes of HECs.

The following perspectives will be scrutinised in the process:

- a view of modern society as a functionally differentiated society without a central ethical/moral perspective;
- a perspective of the status of bioethical issues for achieving public and political consensus;
- an empirical perspective of the real-time practice of committee-supported ethics which, in contrast to the academic reflection practice of the ethical work of the concept, must find the means to generate ethical decisions and reasons under different conditions involving incomplete information, limited time, cooperation constraints, participation pressure and goal-oriented discourse.

Hospital ethics committees as a typical example

Ethical forms of reflection are always linked to certain *images of human beings*, from which the status of the particular speaker's position is derived. In this case also, the perspective of our research does not become involved in the reasons for, or the invention of human images. It views rather the problem of human images empirically by inquiring after the image of the subject of the ethical decision. This is usually the self-responsible, more or less autonomous and at least accountable individual, who, in the Western tradition, may be called the subject because they are equipped with a kind of internal infinity that offers sufficient *requisite variety* to make the accountability credible. A perspective of the actual practice of ethical decision-making in organisations raises doubts as to whether these are the type of people actually making the decisions. It seems much more to be constellations of actors propelled by the dynamics of an institutional context that gives rise to speaker positions, whose practical cooperation and organisational pressures assign a curiously singular dynamic to ethical decision-making. In addition to this, one will find, for instance in the communication between professionals and semi-professionals or between professionals and clients (e.g., doctors and patients) that asymmetrical positions become established which cannot be explained away as a rational basis for communication, neither with goodwill nor with the philosophical norms of 'eye-level' encounter (Maynard 1991; Saake 2003; Nassehi 2004).

Even the medical-critical communications, for example, in HECs, have become aware of just how rewarding the theoretical switch of the systems theory to communication is, in other words to the issue of generating order through the creation of connectivity (Luhmann 1995: 137–8).

The concept of HECs comes from the USA (Lilje 1995; Engelhardt 1999). It is centred on the idea of an interdisciplinary debate about the best medical therapy and an overall concern over the patients' needs (Siegler 1986; Michel 1993: 80). In the outcome, these committees produced a special bureaucratic process of including different status groups of employees as well as non-employees (laypersons, patients) (Sulilatu 2008). There has been a German debate about these institutions since the late 1990s, and since then there exist first experiences with this form of ethical speaking in hospitals. The first results of research on HECs were quite pessimistic because HECs did not seem to meet the expectations of an adequate ethical decision-making process.

Our own research is not focused on the adequacy of ethical speaking in a substantial or normative manner. Beyond that, our research is interested in the practice of German HECs and the ethical dimension of this practice. This research project at the universities of Munich and Göttingen (Germany) was supported by the DFG (Deutsche Forschungsgemeinschaft; German Research Foundation). The interviews cited in the following have been conducted in German at German hospitals.[1]

The methodological foundation is a functionalistic method, which seeks out the reference problem of sentences. Empirical data are understood as solutions for problems in so far as they react to problems of a certain context. We are looking for repeated sentences and read them as evidence for their viability. This viability is then interpreted in reference to a special context and its function (Nassehi 2003a; Nassehi and Saake 2002).

The first quote we present stems from an interview with a patients' representative.

Well, the main problems are communication. Communication, is, let's say, let's start with the doctors, well they're, it's always the patients who ask the questions, and it is always the doctor who answers, and it's never actually clear what it's all about. That the doctors don't have enough time is also clear. It's very much on the communication level that it doesn't work. Of course, there are patients who are unhappy in themselves, who you can never really calm down, but for the most part it's through the discussions we have, that we can usually solve it ourselves, the problem. We have cases where the communication between the doctor and patient is so disrupted that we conduct mediation discussions in our rooms, in other words we invite the patient, and we invite the doctor involved, and try in a small group usually with Mrs. [name] from Quality Management, we try to carry out mediation.

(E-WG-6: 41–53)

The major aspect here is not what is being reported, as that seems quite clear. Far more decisive is the fact that it is being reported and that it seems so clear. The patient's representative is communicating about the communication and makes clear that the practice in a hospital is such that different perspectives confront each other, different presents and different practices which cannot be brought together through the expertise of the doctor but only by discussing the communication itself can insights be gained.

An oncologist formulates a similar view when considering the difference between medical and nursing perspectives:

> I think that this is the cause of the problems. If, well, since eh, it can be forecast, that the nurses for instance will come, we've already had that, there on Monday, you know, this poor communication, the nurse, who did not find out, why what was done, for example. You see there is obviously a communication problem again. No one tells them, although I did in fact raise the subject later, certainly, it is difficult, whether we should make these decisions together, it would be a good idea. But of course it would have to be such, the decision, that the doctor could stick up for it because he must take the responsibility in front of [name of the head of the medical department]. If we haven't got this consensus, eh, then he has to like make the decision alone, against the rest of the world if necessary. But, when they did talk about it, then the others at least knew what the reasons where for his decision. Now whether that is subjective, justifiable or unjustifiable pressures or whatever, but at least they knew how the decision came to be made. And then I believe that the nursing staff can deal with it far more easily, even with decisions that they don't have to make themselves.
>
> (E-W-12: 848–62)

In this case too, the discussion of the crisis diagnosis does not focus on whether the decision was right or wrong, but exclusively on the order-generating role of communication. Simply the fact *that* communication took place seems to be the decisive point here, not the deliberate dispelling of differences in perspectives. The issue is one of respect and recognition, and in this respect it appears that the power structure and the asymmetry between the professional and client or semi-professional roles are being hidden behind their communicative relativisation, without of course completely disappearing.

At a first glance, this practice of ethical communication might appear to be a democratisation of decision-making processes – democratisation in respect of a participation of all concerned actors with the aim to come to a common or commonly legitimised solution. This might point to an ethical perspective such as the discourse ethics of Jürgen Habermas (1990a, 1990b). What can most definitely be observed is the *demand* for symmetrisation and democratisation. The whole of the debate about clinical ethics committees and clinical ethical consultancy is in the end determined by such demands; even when the prime objective is not the solving of all decision-making problems, the aim is at least to relativise the medical power monopoly in favour of an internal democratisation. But, in fact, it is exactly these democratisation demands that facilitate the asymmetrical decisions.

The function of democracy is misunderstood when it is seen as a generator of consensus (Luhmann 1979; Nassehi 2002, 2003b). The democratic programme binds the holder of power (in other words, the 'sovereign' or superior) to stick to his own decisions, even at the price of deferring his own insight to that which has been asserted. Democracy does not prove itself through consensus but rather through the tolerance of dissent and at times through the transfer of dissent experiences to the consensus of what is to be accepted now. The political formula of 'democracy' as the central self-descriptive instance of modern political formats thus enables the people who are affected to be stylised as the decision-makers. In this sense, democracy protects the powerful from the powerless rather than the reverse – and in this sense it is attractive to extend the programme formula of democratisation not just to political areas in the narrower sense but to society as a whole, knowing full well that almost nothing in modern society can be traced back to a binding democratic decision. No decision at all, on economic figures or scientific truth, on artistic styles or love, not even on what is visible in the mass media and most definitely not the relevance of religious content, is made *democratically*. The programme formula is so attractive for this very reason alone. It throws up questions of legitimation, not in the sense that legitimation will be *found* but in the sense that the function of the question in the continuing and normalising of what in the end must always be seen as *irrational* solutions.

This also applies to day-to-day hospital politics, as can be seen in our two illuminating examples of the patient representative and the oncologist. The reference to the *democratisation* of day-to-day hospital life aims not only at democratising decision-making but also at breaking the organisational/medical routine in favour of the power *circle* which lends the medical position its *authority* in the first place. The *informed consent* does nothing other than this either.[2] It forms an interruption in the routine of the *informed* decision-making process. The *competence* dimension of the decision-making process is thus interrupted by the *social* dimension of *consent*, in other words by an *individual decision*.

Symmetricising forms of communication serve then, almost ironically, to create mutual recognition of the speakers' incommensurability by increasing their respective authenticity. We use the term 'authenticity' to demonstrate that it is the person that matters rather than the persons' arguments. Authenticity in this understanding is a specific communicative tool to reprieve communication from the explosive and dividing potential of different arguments. Authenticity as a communicative resource is able to locate different speakers on eye level – beyond their professional and social origin and at least temporarily beyond different statuses. This, in this sense of 'democratising' practice, is indeed the basis for the peaceful coexistence of incommensurable practices, which thus become commensurable. The different speaker positions of the doctor, the patient representative, the patient and other speakers can, through mutual recognition, perpetuate the recognition of *their own* practice formats and thus act as if they were all involved in a mutual reference system. That is what probably can be signified as polyphony, with regard to what we have said in our introduction: as the occurrence of different voices and sounds in organisations. It is exactly for this reason that the conversion *communication* is being engineered even in the self-reflection of practice.

As will now be demonstrated, the idea of discourse in particular feeds on a high level of trust in the order-generating power of communication, as manifested in the institutionalised form of clinical ethics committees. It is from this perspective (we are only interested in connectivity from a systems-theory perspective[3]) that new perspectives emerge on a research issue which can be summarised as follows: the function of HECs is at best unclear and at worst does not exist at all. Approaches to this subject begin with the findings that it is obviously not about concrete decisions (Michel 1993: 80) and not about a consensus (Moreno 1988: 428). Instead, the process itself and the consensus about the process (Moreno 1988: 428), or something like a 'narrative approach' (Brody 1999: 50; Poirier 1999: 35) themselves represent a reasonable meeting because

> [w]hile it is unlikely that an ethics committee would ever explicitly address the moral fragmentation of Western or American culture in the midst of a case review, there are attitudes that committee members might readily strike that do reflect these subtle cultural conditions. I would like to comment on two: a tendency towards ethical skepticism and relativism, and a tendency to consign ethical matters to one's 'private life'.
>
> (Blake 1992: 7)

What sounds here like an attempt to gain something positive out of a failed experiment is due to the tone of voice which in the ethical sense is a solution in itself. The style of Richard Moskowitz is very similar:

> It is therefore inevitable that serious ethical conflicts should occur within the hospital. The amazing thing is that HECs have succeeded so well with them, while their parent hospitals are often powerless to resolve issues of far lesser difficulty and importance. Their healing function clearly has to do with their ability to articulate moral values which are generally recognised and adhered to throughout the hospital community. But it also implies a commitment to broad and faithful representation of the diversity of interests and viewpoints in the hospital and the

community at large, and to a process of dialogue and mutual respect in an attempt to reconcile them when they disagree.

(Moskowitz 1989: 36)

While the opponents of such an approach can plausibly accept criticism of the procedure and promise a better future for the HECs if they professionalise their procedures (Wolf 1992, 1993; Hoffmann 1994; Hayes 1995), in the following section we would like to turn the argumentation around. The HECs' apparent lack of function is not the problem but rather the solution in so far as under the special conditions a form of address has developed that breaks precisely with the classic expectations of functionality, consistency and professionalism. It is a practical symptom of an organisation that cannot use monophonic styles of self-description any more. While the vanishing point of a philosophical discussion always offers the possibility of agreement, group discussions on the subject of ethics, according to the statements made by participants of HECs, seem in the first place to be especially suitable to practically mediating the experience of difference.

A patient representative, also in the HEC, who had just begun her contribution, formulated it in a very similar manner to that of the ethical consultation (Saake and Kunz 2006), saying that she found it very positive to experience in the discussion that other people could see things differently:

> Well, we also had the experience at congresses that cases were presented on which concrete work had been done, and that had been helpful to someone, because other people saw it quite differently, for instance. You got the chance to see the variety. I think that is very important, and I also think it is important that we, now in this group, naturally deal anonymously with cases that occur with us. It is, it has: something to be said for it too. So I think of course the case studies do help somewhat.
>
> (E-WG-6: 516–21)

Different ways of looking at things translate into opposite opinions, and their expression, especially in the committee, can gain in importance against the backdrop of opinions as is clear from the statement made by a chief physician.

I: Hm, what do you wish to express specifically to the ethics committee? How would you describe it?

B: That's just another general formulation that doesn't say anything to me, eh, I try, the things, that are being discussed simply, with what I think, what appears to me to be right, so that I can contribute something when other opinions are being aired.

(E-HT-13: 218–23)

A surgeon reports about the effects the many ways of viewing an issue have on his own perspective:

B: I simply say now what I feel, what is good for me, if the discussion with people who simply have another way of looking at things and who view and discuss the issue in an open discussion round, evaluation round, simply from different perspectives. That means, I listen happily when a Pastor Kern, or a Ms. Hauck, or a Ms. Lustig, or a Doctor Stein, or simply from –, or the nursing personnel, just simply in the situation, you see? The non-medical side for once, how does someone see it who sees it from the outside or from another position, how is the issue viewed, what values have a massive importance and what values do we not really take any notice of?

That means, the thing about bodily injury, that we perform every day, with the consent of our patients of course –, make, is –, we make it just something normal that we do every day. And then, for example, a Ms. Hauck comes along, who became involved in the discussion about the patient who was given a PEG [percutaneous endoscopic gastrostomy] without her consent and asks how … how shocking, or how extreme this reaction also seems from someone who sees it really as it is, yes as bodily injury but with what a degree of emotionality, of sentimentality it was brought into the discussion by someone, emotionality that we ourselves are not aware of. Yes I find the whole thing is an expansion of my horizons, yes, what I say ethically morally, but also my thinking horizon.

II: Mhm. That probably doesn't make it easier as a doctor, does it?

B: Yes it does make it easier.

II: It does?

B: Yes. It makes it easier, because you can recognise why someone reacts with fear in this situation, I erm, I can recognise, then I feel again as a normal person, as a human being who gets into such a situation and says, OK, so like now on the intensive-care ward with one patient, I can understand the difficult situation people find themselves in, who normally have nothing to do with medicine in this borderline situation, who simply feel overwhelmed, literally steamrollered, you see?

(E-WG-15: 134–63)

By acknowledging other perspectives, the 'normality' of one's own view becomes relativised, one's own perspective is recognisable as one *perspective* among others. It is not the matter-of-fact things of the everyday working world which should form the basis of the situation evaluation, the asymmetry is pushed much more in the direction of a non-medical, normal perspective which must then be understood and taken on board. Accordingly, a *good* participant in the discourse (in other words, a participant who acts as one in the discourse) is characterised less by arguing consistently over a period of time than by being flexible and showing their ability to change perspectives. There will be more on this later.

The idea of interdisciplinarity, to which the composition of the ethics committees from different professions seems to be geared, appears from a discourse perspective to be a necessary prerequisite to allow a free play of the good reasons (Capron 1985). In the context of the ethics committees, however, it loses some of its instrumental character, and even the production of a multiplicity of viewpoints appears to be the aim of an ethical discussion rather than being just a partial victory.

Against this horizon, being of different opinions appears almost entirely unproblematic:

> That too is an experience for me, to ask someone about his autonomy and so on, it's been many years, but it was a decisive point for me, so to speak, I have my opinion, the person, the person affected had a different opinion and we still get on although our opinions are the exact opposite! Well, not exactly opposite, but very contrary. And I believe that when you deal with each other like that, then I believe that you can even allow ethical problems to stand, at least if people do not explode and emotionally eh completely decompensate.
>
> (E-WG-15: 663–71)

Having another opinion is not only not a problem, it is actually seen as a solution since we are only dealing with *opinions*. The productivity of the discourse is measured not according to how far it contributes to a consensus but to how much it contributes to producing different speakers.

Seen in terms of social history, one cannot imagine a form of society in which a 'natural state' would tolerate symmetrical speaker positions in the long term. A situation where everyone is allowed to have their say – even should have their say – is initially a highly unlikely social situation, and the dyed-in-the wool discourse theoreticians would not accept that the idea of a power-free discourse was anything other than an ideal, a theoretical claim rather than an empirical description.[4] However, it has been observed that in the ethics committees a discourse has become established in which the speaker positions can no longer be legitimately limited. One also sees that situations in which speakers get the chance to speak have to be repeatedly re-established.[5]

The descriptions of a former doctor and member of the ethics committee illustrate the consequences of this particular type of openness for potential speakers in the committee:

> And I must say, my idea was, well, when I allowed myself, eh, eh, for example with someone who wished to speak, a dialogue ensued, and I was warned again and again that there was a speaker list, but it had only been my intention to clarify some concepts with him. So,

something was said, perhaps a term such as 'self-determination', or 'enlightenment', or like, oh I don't know, 'truth' or something like that, and it was my intention to ask what was meant by these terms, in order to make it clearer for the group what was being said. Because if I just let a discussion like that run, so that everyone around the table just presents his statement then in the end I just have a collection of statements in which the same term may be used seven times but is probably used differently seven times.

(E-WG-12: 231–41)

The reference to a speakers' list in the discourse is apparently very difficult to ignore, which is why the clarification of and agreement on terms took second place to the right to be heard – to the regret of the interviewee. From the position of the sociological observers this cannot be criticised; of far more sociological interest are the consequences for the discussion of this behaviour if this approach leads to a 'collection of statements' which will then have to be dealt with in later practice.

Just how much discursive decision-making is interpreted as a symmetrising event can be seen in the idea of being on a par with the other members, which has to be learnt in the hierarchically structured hospital organisation:

So we try now and again to get a discussion round going, so that everyone can learn how to discuss and to get over inhibitions when speaking to the consultant, and the consultant could start looking a bit less arrogant when speaking to a nurse, well all these things, and if, I believe if it had been practiced a little over the long term – you can't do it in a year, then another type of everyday behavior would become normal, and the nursing staff because they would have the space where they could speak in a certain manner, and then they would be able to do it a bit more on the ward, if the situation allowed it, but these are long-term projects that would take years.

(E-HB-1: 44–53)

In the view of this doctor, a successful discussion requires competent speakers capable of contributing to the discussion. For this to happen, different persons must see themselves in the first place as speakers in order to position themselves as speakers. This should not be misinterpreted as a reflexive or transparent use of the own position. To present oneself as a speaker means to utilise the structure of this specific situation in which different positions, statuses and arguments become deconstructed as different speaker positions, whereas the difference of professional perspectives becomes disarmed by the authentic construction of speaker positions. A lack of this competence is found particularly among the nursing staff who are, however, supposed to learn this in the protected space of the ethics committee, to present themselves as speakers and thus be able to stand up to the consultant in the future.

Consequences for ethics, or, the ruse of ethical reason

At the end of our discussion we would like to briefly consider the consequences of our results for ethical theory and for a theory of polyphonic or better: polycontextural organisations. Organisational practices such as those of hospitals, government policy, advertising, the suitable treatment of animals, of investment decisions, cannot be conditioned or programmed with such new philosophical-scientific labels as medical ethics, political ethics, ethics in advertising, animal ethics or industrial ethics and economic ethics. In the case of medical ethics, sure enough it can clearly be seen that there has been a marked ethical sensitisation of problems. And we believe that we can say normatively with our results that HECs are indeed ethically significant, that is to say in so far as they create a form that meets one of the expectations of a culture accustomed to symmetrical communication, even in organisations which in the end functionally serve the suspension of symmetry requirements. How else are organisations to deal with the multiplicity of speaker positions than by establishing islands inside the organisations where these may be visible *as speaker positions* – this is one of our results.

Ethical theory must, however, still continue to ask itself how it can be in a position to *shorten* ethical arguments, i.e. to make sure that it at least offers criteria or procedures to distinguish right from wrong. Whether (as in the case of) we are talking about the discourse on evolving values and their integrative power (Joas 2001), whether the discourse of the ethical potential of the language can be seen as a basis on which morally integrated action coordination can be emphasised (Habermas 1990a), whether it can be cultivated in the sense of Rawls' justice as a basic category of adequate socialisation (Rawls 1971) or in particulate communicative liberalism criticism, limited to patriotic universalisms (Sandel 1982; Taylor 1992; Etzioni, 1993), whether a minimal morality compatible with differentiated modernity can be shaped in contrast to the communitaristic revitalisation of Durkheimianism, as practised by Gertrud Nunner-Winkler (2001), for instance, whether reference is made to theoretical coherence and embedding in a structural rationality in the sense of a theory of rationality (Nida-Rümelin 2000) or whether a general humanity is posited as the moral yardstick of the social as with Martha Nussbaum in an Aristotelian-essentialist sense (Nussbaum 1995), the discourse always takes the form that it on the one hand still emphasises the integrative force of moral judgement while on the other hand shortening the argumentative possibilities. Scientific ethics is not possible without such a shortening algorithm. It must at least demonstrate an intuition of a true or right ethical perception and its rationality to be ethically meaningful. Taking this as a presumption, the ethical practice in the HECs contradicts this diametrically, since it is exactly the opposite that succeeds here: arguments, speakers and reasons are produced and multiplied, and *in this* and *only in this* is the ethical sense of communication revealed in practice. It is particularly interesting from a sociological perspective because it is only this perspective that can see how such locations develop for the special form of 'ethical' speaking, without itself falling into the pattern of ethical speaking. To all others it will only appear to be evidence of the lack of function of HECs, who then somehow rescue themselves 'ethically' by finding it positive to get into discussion with each other.

The consequences of these results reach much further. They are an almost symbolic expression of the 'society of presents' (Nassehi 2006, 2011), i.e. a society that is able to disconnect presences and to do without a strong idea of integration. In that sense, this description of modernity is a radically post-Parsonian systems-theoretical description. Our empirical results show that HECs are sociologically more significant than they may first appear. Two things can be observed in HECs: on the one hand, the recognition of the incommensurability of different forms of practice and reflection perspectives are celebrated. HECs deal with the structural impossibility of generating a total perspective from different professional and practical perspectives. In contrast, the functional meaning of HECs appears to be to accomplish communicatively and to be decidedly able to forbear the use of such a perspective.

In ethical theory, this experience (in the German-speaking world at least) has been embedded in the incontrovertible prominence of the discourse ethics of Karl-Otto Apel (1990) and Jürgen Habermas (1990b) (see also Kettner 1996, 1999). It reflects ethically and philosophically what can be practically empirically observed: the practical efficacious substance of the ethical committee does not consist of good and better reasons but of more and more authentic speakers. For reasons of space, we cannot show here how this is reflected in the philosophical-ethical discourse. Finally, we would like to point out that our empirical results have far broader sociological significance than simply in reference to HECs.

The ability of modern societies to disconnect perspectives, different conditions of success, different logics, different ways of thinking, different situations, in this sense: different presences from each other can be observed in the practice of the HECs. What is decided in HECs and what commitments, fictions of consensus and common papers are generated does not in any way condition clinical practice. The present of the committee meetings differs from the present of clinical decision-making practice on the wards. HECs learn mentalities in order to avoid mediating these presents. They thus form both a culturalising and, therefore, an interlocking recognition of different perspectives: medical, religious, nursing, patient, ethical, economic and other perspectives are communicated without being mediated. Care is taken that they can be spoken about authentically. HECs do not take the drama out of the pressure of decision-making. Like all organisations, organisations in health care are decision machines (Nassehi 2005b). But they do take the drama out of the incommensurability of decision-making presents and generate a space within the clinic in which other rules apply than those that apply in the clinic outside of the committee.

To a certain extent, HECs channel culturalising interruptions and appoint speakers who are not explicitly found on the committees even when the 'human beings' involved on the ward and the committee are possibly the same, they are not the same 'persons' (Nassehi 2007). The HEC reflects how modern society disintegrates into presents in the manner of a functionally differentiated society which does not treat its incommensurability from their perspective as a problem or fault but rather, in fact, as a potential.

A technical term which is able to describe the societal basis for empirical studies of ethics is 'polycontexurality'. For example, Til Jansen and Werner Vogd (2013) use this term in the context of organisation theory, which stems from Gotthard Günther (1979). Günther has used this term to show that every perspective on the world is the function of its own perspective. He calls this perspective a *contexture* in difference to a *context*, which is only a special kind of environment or a precondition of a perspective. A contexture for Günther is the perspective itself, which cannot become denied by itself. But an observer can see that different perspectives are bound to different contextures. Günther disputes the law of the excluded middle, which was the basic law of the Aristotelian thinking. He shows that every perspective has its own ontological basis, but he also can show that different perspectives produce different ontological shapes of the world. This is what he calls polycontexturality.

Niels Åkerstrøm Andersen thus talks about 'polyphonic organisations' in order to show that 'in effect a large number of new organisations have become aesteticised, politicised, and educationalised' (2001). This, he asserts, is a problem most of all for managers who have to take into consideration many different accounts at the same time that develop in the same organisation without hierarchies: 'social accounts, ethical accounts, knowledge accounts, employee accounts etc.' (Åkerstrøm Andersen 2001). As we have stated at the beginning of our argumentation, we cannot follow Akerstrøm Åndersen when he asserts this to be a new phenomenon. Apart from the all-too-generalised assertion that the different functional logics would be handled without hierarchies, we have doubts about the diagnosis of a new perspectivism.

The difference of perspectives is a phenomenon known at least since the Renaissance. As we have mentioned in the introduction to our paper, organisations themselves can be seen as techniques of dealing with the difference of perspectives. Modernisation was always paralleled by the occurrence of organisations and of organisation arrangements to make the difference of perspectives expectable and practically manageable. Generally, management is a practice to deal with different perspectives which have to be interconnected or at least have to find ways of a continuing coexistence. This can be called the basic character of societal modernity since the end of the eighteenth century. What is really new is that nowadays organisations become confronted with their different perspectives and challenged by demands stemming from outside of their own practice. To come to terms with this they develop new forms of communication strategies.

The ethicisation of practices is one of these strategies. As we tried to show, the ruse of ethical reason is its ability to deal with different speakers without harmonising or reconciling the different perspectives. Modern observers of differences seem to be used to the experience that the world has different shapes and meanings. The dislocation of ethical reasons to the ethical speaking of different perspectives is a sign of a society that operates radically as a polycontextural system.

We call this, in systems-theory terms, a *society of presents*, in which the continuity of a total perspective gives way to concrete presents (Nassehi 2003a, 2004, 2005a, 2006, 2011). A modern, functionally differentiated society can only be in possession of political or ethically effective self-descriptions that aim at the whole and wish to produce the continuity of an integrated society showing solidarity, and which has split off from other presents – just as the HECs have broken off from standard hospital practice but use the different speaker positions that draw on the different routines of societal self-description established by functional differentiation. In this respect, it is in fact the HECs apparent *lack of function* which is their true *functional* feature. One can learn from the example of HECs that a modern society with a strict interconnection of its instances is unthinkable and that society's modern moral and functional disintegration is not to be treated as a structural defect. On the contrary, this is the basic structure and asset of modern social conditions, in which the interruption of interdependencies can be regarded as the source of repeatedly new forms of interdependence and of the recombination of possibilities. In our perspective, the sociology of modernity has known this from its very beginning but has concealed this experience by theories of integration and overcoming differences. In that respect, sociology often is akin to the basic intuition of ethics, at least of theoretical or philosophical ethics. But our empirical results of ethical practice in a body like a HEC show the ethical potential of this practice is diametrically opposed to the basic intuitions of the formation of ethical theory with its attempt to integrate the different and plural. And one can always learn from this, which is just where we started with our thesis: ethics is only a scientific discipline, disconnected from practices that give themselves the same name.

Notes

1 The qualitative field research in this DFG-funded project was situated in four German hospitals, concentrating on four HECs. The database consists of sixty-four interviews and seventy-four observation protocols.
2 See Tom L. Beauchamp and Ruth Faden (1995) for more details on the emergence and criticism of this term.
3 The focus on connectivity means that we look at the conditions under which communication can continue. The concept of connectivity is undetermined enough to describe how different conditions of further communications emerge empirically.

4 See Habermas (1984/1987) in general and Kettner (1996, 1999) with regard to HECs.
5 It is quite remarkable that such expectations of a symmetrical communication style can only be achieved within the context of an organisation, one level of creating social order, where one always seems to recognise the asymmetry. Interestingly, self-descriptions of such discourse trust more than anything else in interaction, which, as another level of the social creation of order is also full of asymmetries, can always only be addressed sequentially and can always only focus on one subject at a time (Luhmann 1975).

References

Åkerstrøm Andersen, N. (2001) *Polyphonic Organizations*, MPP Working Paper 13/2001.

Apel, K.-O. (1990) 'Is the Ethics of the Ideal Communication Community a Utopia? On the Relationship between Ethics, Utopia, and the Critique of Utopia', in S. Benhabib and F. Dallmayr (eds.), *The Communicative Ethics Controversy*, Cambridge, Mass.: MIT Press, pp. 23–59.

Beauchamp, T. L. and R. Faden (1995) 'Meaning and Elements of Informed Consent', in W. Reich (ed.), *Encyclopedia of Bioethics*, New York: Simon & Schuster Macmillan, pp. 1238–41.

Blake, D. C. (1992) 'The Hospital Ethics Committee: Health Care's Moral Conscience or White Elephant?', *Hastings-Center-Report*, 22 (1): 6–11.

Brody, H. (1999) 'Narrative Ethics and Institutional Impact', *HEC Forum*, 11 (1): 46–51.

Capron, A. M. (1985) 'Legal Perspectives on Institutional Ethics Committees', *Journal of College and University Law*, 11 (4): 417–31.

Engelhardt, H. T. Jr. (1999) 'Healthcare Ethics Committees: Re-Examining Their Social and Moral Functions', *HEC Forum*, 11 (2): 87–100.

Etzioni, A. (1993) *The Spirit of Community: Rights, Responsibilities, and the Communitarian Agenda*, New York: Crown Publishers.

Günther, G. (1979) 'Life as Poly-Contexturality', in *Beiträge zur Grundlegung einer operationsfähigen Dialektik, Band 2*, Hamburg: Meiner, pp. 283–306.

Habermas, J. (1984) *The Theory of Communicative Action*, 2 vols, Boston, Mass.: Beacon Press.

——(1990a) *Moral Consciousness and Communicative Action*, Cambridge, Mass.: MIT Press.

——(1990b) 'Discourse Ethics: Notes on a Program of Philosophical Justification', in S. Benhabib and F. Dallmayr (eds.), *The Communicative Ethics Controversy*, Cambridge, Mass.: MIT Press, pp. 43–115.

Hayes, G. J. (1995) 'Ethics Committees: Group Process Concerns and the Need for Research', *Cambridge Quarterly of Health Care Ethics*, 4 (1): 83–91.

Hoffmann, D. E. (1994) 'Case Consultation: Paying Attention to Process', in S. Spicker (ed.), *The Healthcare Ethics Committee Experience: Selected Readings from HEC Forum*, Malabar, Fla.: Krieger Publishing Company, pp. 257–64.

Jansen, T. and W. Vogd (2013) 'Polykontexturale Verhältnisse: disjunkte Rationalitäten am Beispiel von Organisationen', *Zeitschrift für theoretische Soziologie*, 1 (2): 82–97.

Joas, H. (2001) *The Genesis of Values*, Chicago, Ill.: University of Chicago Press.

Keown, J. (2005) 'Mr Marty's Muddle: A Superficial and Selective Case for Euthanasia in Europe', *Journal of Medical Ethics*, 32 (1): 29–33.

Kettner, M. (1996) 'Discourse Ethics and Health Care Ethics Committees', *Jahrbuch für Recht und Ethik*, 4: 249–72.

——(1999) 'Discourse Ethics: A Novel Approach to Moral Decision Making', *International Journal of Bioethics*, 10 (3): 29–36.

Lilje, Christian (1995) *Klinische,ethics consultation' in den USA: Hintergründe, Denkstile und Praxis*, Stuttgart: Enke.

Luhmann, N. (1975) 'Interaktion, Organisation, Gesellschaft', in *Soziologische Aufklärung 2: Aufsätze zur Theorie der Gesellschaft*, Opladen: Westdeutscher Verlag, pp. 9–20.

——(1979) *Trust and Power*, Chichester: John Wiley.

——(1995) *Social Systems*, Stanford, Calif.: Stanford University Press.

——(1996) 'The Sociology of the Moral and Ethics', *International Sociology*, 11 (1): 27–36.

——(1998) *Observations on Modernity*, Stanford, Calif.: Stanford University Press.

——(2002) *Theories of Distinction: Redescribing the Description of Modernity*, edited by William Rasch, Stanford, Calif.: Stanford University Press.

Maynard, D. (1991) 'Interaction and Asymmetry in Clinical Discourse', *American Journal of Sociology*, 97 (2): 448–95.

Michel, V. (1993) 'The Ethics Committee as a "Community of Concern": A Reflection on the Accountability of Bioethics Committees and Consultants', in S. Spicker (ed.), *The Healthcare Ethics Committee Experience: Selected Readings from HEC Forum*, Malabar, Fla.: Krieger, pp. 76–80.

Moreno, J. D. (1988) 'Ethics by Committee: The Moral Authority of Consensus', *Journal of Medicine and Philosophy*, 13 (4): 411–32.

Moskowitz, R. (1989) 'Hospital Ethics Committees: The Healing Function', in S. Spicker (ed.), *The Healthcare Ethics Committee Experience: Selected Readings from HEC Forum*, Malabar, Fla.: Krieger, pp. 32–8.

Nassehi, A. (2001) 'Religion und Moral: Zur Säkularisierung der Moral und der Moralisierung der Religion in der modernen Gesellschaft', in M. Krüggeler and G. Pickel (eds.), *Religion und Moral*, Opladen: Westdeutscher Verlag, pp. 21–38.

——(2002) 'Politik des Staates oder Politik der Gesellschaft? Kollektivität als Problemformel des Politischen', in K. U. Hellmann and R. Schmalz-Bruns (eds.), *Die Politik der Gesellschaft: Beiträge zu Luhmanns Theorie des politischen Systems*, Frankfurt: Suhrkamp, pp. 38–59.

——(2003a) *Geschlossenheit und Offenheit: Studien zur Theorie der modernen Gesellschaft*, Frankfurt: Suhrkamp.

——(2003b) 'Der Begriff des Politischen und die doppelte Normativität der 'soziologischen' Moderne', in A. Nassehi and M. Schroer (eds.), *Der Begriff des Politischen*, Baden-Baden: Nomos, pp. 133–69.

——(2004) 'Formen der Vergesellschaftung des Sterbeprozesses'. Paper presented at a public symposium of the Nationaler Ethikrat (German National Ethics Council).

——(2005a) 'Society', in A. Harrington, B. L. Marshall and H.-P. Müller (eds.), *Encyclopedia of Social Theory*, London and New York: Routledge, pp. 436–41.

——(2005b) 'Organizations as Decision Machines: Niklas Luhmann's Theory of Organized Social Systems', in C. Jones and R. Munro (eds.), *Contemporary Organization Theory*, Oxford: Blackwell, pp. 178–91.

——(2006) *Der soziologische Diskurs der Moderne*, Frankfurt: Suhrkamp.

——(2007) 'The Person as an Effect of Communication', in S. Maasen (ed.), *On Willing Selves: Neoliberal Politics Vis-à-Vis the Neuroscientific Challenge*, Basingstoke: Palgrave Macmillan, pp. 100–20.

——(2011) *Gesellschaft der Gegenwarten: Studien zur Theorie der modernen Gesellschaft II*, Frankfurt: Suhrkamp.

Nassehi, A. and I. Saake (2002) 'Kontingenz: Methodisch verhindert oder beobachtet? Ein Beitrag zur Methodologie der qualitativen Sozialforschung', *Zeitschrift für Soziologie*, 31 (1): 66–86.

Nida-Rümelin, J. (2000) 'Rationality: Coherence and Structure', in J. Nida-Rümelin and W. Spohn (eds.), *Rationality, Rules, and Structure*, Dordrecht: Kluwer Academic Publishers, pp. 1–16.

Nunner-Winkler, G. (2001) 'Devices for Identity Maintenance in Modern Society', in A. van Harskamp and A. W. Musschenga (eds.), *The Many Faces of Individualism*, Leuven: Peeters, pp. 197–224.

Nussbaum, M. C. (1995) 'Aristotle on Human Nature and the Foundations of Ethics', in J. E. J. Altham and Ross Harrison (eds.), *World, Mind, and Ethics: Essays on the Ethical Philosophy of Bernard Williams*, Cambridge: Cambridge University Press, pp. 86–131.

Poirier, S. (1999) 'Voice: Structure, Politics, and Values in the Medical Narrative', *HEC Forum*, 11 (1): 27–37.

Rawls, J. (1971) *A Theory of Justice*, Cambridge, Mass.: Harvard University Press.

Reamer, F. G. (1987) 'Ethics Committees in Social Work', *Social Work*, 32 (3): 188–92.

Saake, I. (2003) 'Die Performanz des Medizinischen: Zur Asymmetrie der Arzt-Patienten-Intertaktion', *Soziale Welt*, 54 (4): 429–61.

Saake, I., and D. Kunz (2006) 'Von Kommunikation über Ethik zu "ethischer Sensibilisierung": Symmetrisierungsprozess in diskursiven Verfahren', *Zeitschrift für Soziologie*, 35 (1): 41–56.

Sandel, M. J. (1982) *Liberalism and the Limits of Justice*, Cambridge: Cambridge University Press.

Siegler, Mark (1986) 'Ethics Committees: Decisions by Bureaucracy', *Hastings Center Report*, 16 (3): 22–4.

Sulilatu, S. (2008) 'Klinische Ethik-Komitees als Verfahren der Entbürokratisierung?' in I. Saake and W. Vogd (eds.), *Moderne Mythen der Medizin: Studien zur organisierten Krankenbehandlung*, Wiesbaden: VS Verlag, pp. 285–306.

Sureau, C. (1995) 'Medical Deresponsibilization', *Journal of Assisted Reproduction and Genetics*, 12 (8): 552–8.

Taylor, C. (1992) *Sources of the Self: The Making of the Modern Identity*, Cambridge, Mass.: Harvard University Press.

van den Daele, W. (2001a) 'Von moralischer Kommunikation zur Kommunikation über Moral. Reflexive Distanz in diskursiven Verfahren', *Zeitschrift für Soziologie*, 30 (1): 4–22.

——(2001b) 'Gewissen, Angst und radikale Reform: Wie starke Ansprüche an die Technikpolitik in diskursiven Arenen schwach werden', in G. Simonis, R. Martinsen and T. Saretzki (eds.), *Politik und Technik: Analysen zum Verhältnis von technologischem Wandel am Anfang des 21 Jahrhunderts*, Wiesbaden: Westdeutscher Verlag, pp. 476–98.

Wolf, S. M. (1992) 'Due Process in Ethics Committee Case Review', in S. Spicker (ed.), *The Healthcare Ethics Committee Experience: Selected Readings from HEC Forum*, Malabar, Fla.: Krieger, pp. 243–56.

——(1993) 'Toward a Theory of Process', *Law, Medicine and Health Care*, 20 (4): 278–90.

9 Polycontexturality in medical research ethics

Barry Gibson and Jennifer Burr

In this chapter we use the concept of polycontexturality to explore the content of codes of research ethics. We argue that research ethics provides a space in which to bring together often conflicting contextures that enable research to happen. This is in contrast to some views and arguments in sociology and other disciplines that research ethics actually curtail research. For example, research ethics have been perceived as a form of political censorship (Haggerty 2004), as 'unethical' (Dingwall 2006) and as restrictive of research efforts (Wald 2004). Recent history has seen an expansion in the use of codes and governance frameworks for research ethics. Within the United Kingdom (UK), organisations such as the National Health Service (NHS), the research councils (including the Medical Research Council [MRC] and the Economic and Social Research Council [ESRC]) and the universities have engaged in increased communication about ethical conduct during research. They have also developed structures of governance to ensure that ethical reflection takes place during research. The research funding bodies have taken the unprecedented step of stating that future funding will be bound to appropriate structures of research governance. It is now difficult to undertake research involving human participants in the UK that doesn't involve some form of ethical reflection.

The chapter begins with some brief reflections on why Niklas Luhmann might be suitable for analysing ethical controversies. The concept of polycontexturality is key and is introduced through the work of Gotthard Günther, who begins his discussion with the law of the Tertium Non Datur (TND). This notion of polycontexturality is important to Luhmann's systems theory. We go on to use the example of polycontexturality developed by Günther Teubner in his analysis of the changing status of contracting. We then go on to apply this concept in exploring research-ethics documents. Our primary concern is to reveal how the concept of polycontexturality can enable us to explore the 'facts' of ethical communication. Our analysis was informed by the expectation that we should be able to observe not only where contextures of ethical communication successfully shape communication about science but also when such contextures are suspended and why. However, before we start, it is important to also briefly outline some notable moments in the history of scientific research which have resulted in the codification of research ethics.

Background: scientific controversies and the codification of ethical communication

There has been an unfortunate history of controversies in medical research, the most obvious being the Nazi atrocities that resulted in the Declaration of Helsinki. While revelations regarding the abuse of people during medical experiments in the Third Reich are commonly referred to as a pivotal point in the history of codes of research ethics, abuses of prisoners, for example, have not been confined to the Nazi regime. An American clinical trial otherwise known as the Tuskegee study, included 600 low-income African-American males, 400 of whom were injected with syphilis. Participants were not informed about this. Rather, they were told they had a form of 'bad blood'. Even after penicillin became available they were not informed that the condition could be treated. It wasn't until 1972 that the existence of the study was leaked to the general public and caused so much embarrassment that it was terminated. By this time, twenty-eight men had died from syphilis, a further 100 from related complications, forty participants' wives had been infected, and nineteen children had contracted the disease at birth (Panno 2005). Other abuses have occurred, for example, in 1963, doctors injected live cancer cells into elderly debilitated patients in a Jewish chronic-disease hospital in the USA. There is also the case of the US Willowbrook Public School, where intellectually disabled children were injected with hepatitis (Schuklenk 2000).

More recently, in the UK, increasing concern with issues of research ethics has been fuelled by research scandals. The Alder Hey organ scandal came to public attention in the late 1990s when it was discovered that dead children's organs had been collected and stored without parental knowledge and consent. These organs were also treated with appalling disregard; in one instance, glands were given to a pharmaceutical company for research in return for financial donations. A public enquiry revealed that the practice had been going on for decades and yet no one was prosecuted. Consequently, the UK government developed the Human Tissue Act, which now makes strict provision for all activities involving human tissue. The UK's NHS developed its Research Governance Framework in response to the Alder Hey Inquiry. This framework now provides an ethical guide for research conducted in health and social care. The Research Governance Framework has impacted on other areas of research, including universities, which also had to demonstrate that they had implemented a robust means of ensuring ethical review.

It is our contention that this increase in communication about research ethics is worthy of sociological attention beyond that of restriction and censorship. If we are to move towards a sociological understanding of research ethics then we need to find an approach that can enable us to take ethical communication seriously.

Why Luhmann's social-systems theory?

One way to unpick this problem might be to place such forms of communication within a wider theory of society. The approach to systems theory adopted by Niklas Luhmann is arguably one of the most comprehensive and sustained attempts in recent years to develop an explicit theory of society (Moeller 2012). He also adopted the position that *society is communication*.

Niklas Luhmann and ethical communication

A central question about ethical communication relates to the position of norms in society (Luhmann 2008). In order to approach this problem, Luhmann argues that we must first analyse the way facts and norms change their position in different social systems, this includes the discipline of sociology. In the legal system, facts are *ordered according to norms*, but in sociology norms *can be treated as facts*, they are *formulas for contra-factual expectations*. In this sense, norms are not really frustrated by behaviour, they are maintained *despite it*. Sociology, then, should concern itself not with the norms and the fact that they exist but whether or not such norms have success when they are communicated (Luhmann 2008). The instruction here is that we should look to see what norms underpin ethical communication in science and then seek to unpack the degree to which they can guide scientific conduct. There are additional features of Luhmann's perspective on ethics worth noting.

The invention of norms involves a *doubling of reality*. We can distinguish between a norm and whether or not it is adhered to (Luhmann 2008). For Luhmann (2008), the problem modern society confronts is that it cannot rely on this doubling of reality to produce a transcendental principle that can be used as an overarching point of control. Luhmann believed that the project to build a transcendental subject had failed and that modern society describes itself 'poly-contextually' through the help of numerous distinctions (Luhmann 2008). This means that in this society an observer can designate objects and at the same time distinguish themself from these objects.[1] This has the effect of placing them in an unmarked space. In this space, they can observe something but not themselves. It is therefore impossible to achieve an overarching position from which to view society, and any view of society will be partial.

The essential condition of a functionally differentiated society is that it results in multiple points of observation which must be maintained for everyone to access. These change rapidly as systems observe each other. It becomes impossible to have an overarching indispensable set of norms that can help steer society. The internal environment of society is uncontrollable for systems. Systems have to respond to an ever-changing, increasingly complex environment. Although these discussions may well seem quite abstract, they have nonetheless been applied more directly in empirical studies of ethical communication. For example, Nassehi *et al.* (2008) explore how ethical decision-making works in practice in relation to medical ethics committees. Ethical decisions are characterised by the way in which *the final moral claim is limited*. Nassehi *et al.* argue that the final decision taken in such committees 'is the ethical discourse' (2008: 134). Medical ethics committees promote the 'interlocking, recognition of different perspectives' and reflect 'how modern society disintegrates into presents' (Nassehi *et al.* 2008: 153).

More recently, Schirmer and Michailakis (2011) have explored the problems associated with the 'Ethical Platform' in the Swedish welfare state. The 'Ethical Platform' was established to help the system focus on avoiding ascriptive categories for decision-making. In doing so it involved establishing a hierarchy where human dignity was placed as the first and overarching principle for the system. This principle involved the idea that 'all people are of equal value and have the same rights regardless of personal characteristics and functions in society' (Schirmer and Michailakis 2011: 270). The principle was reiterated at every point in relation to the welfare state and was said to have dominated all other principles. The problem with this was that the principle itself was based on a contradiction. You cannot treat everyone equally when you have to set priorities. You have to select someone over and above someone else. In other words, the human-dignity principle has *to be suspended under certain conditions*. Schirmer and Michailakis (2011) demonstrated how the principles of need and solidarity are both used to set boundaries around the dignity principle and in the process provide justifiable reasons for setting the principle aside. But their analysis goes further. Not only are other principles used to condition *and* protect the dignity principle, the rationalities of two different systems play a part in conditioning the principle. The principle of need and the principle of solidarity in some way have a much greater affinity with the medical and political systems respectively. So the conditioning of the dignity principle by the principle of need and solidarity occurs as a consequence of functional differentiation.

The analyses of both Nassehi *et al.* (2008) and Schirmer and Michailakis (2011) demonstrate that there is more to be said about ethical communication than promoting anxiety about ethics as a form of political censorship. In each of the foregoing analyses, the conditioning of norms bears some relationship to the form of functional differentiation. Of particular note is the idea that we live in a polycontextural society.

Polycontexturality and the study of research ethics

The concept of polycontexture in Luhmann's social-systems theory was developed out of the cybernetic approach of Gotthard Günther (1976).[2] Polycontexturality refers to a universe composed of an unlimited number of contextures. Contextures are defined with 'reference to the TND, as a domain the boundaries of which cannot be crossed by processes taking place within the range of the domain' (2004: 5). Günther goes on to state that:

> we are forced to assume that all psychic spaces of living organisms – constitute closed contextures. It is self-evident that the process of thinking taking place within one person cannot be continued into the psychic space of a second person. My thoughts, as mental events, are only mine and nobody else's. A second person may produce the very same thoughts; but they are his and can never be mine.
>
> (Günther 2004: 5)

Günther's (2004) discussion of the principle of TND begins with a discussion of the widest generality of the concept within the idea of being or not being. The TND in this discussion refers to the principle that something either is or it is not, there is nothing in between. Günther goes on to indicate that calling something either being or non-being already presupposes something, a contexture. This widest possible 'contexture' Günther refers to is the ontological 'contexture' or 'contexturality'. He goes a step further and states that '[t]he role that the TND plays with regard to the concept of a contexture indicates that the structure of such a domain can be exhaustively described by a two valued logic' (Günther 2004: 3). Note that in this quotation Günther is indicating that the two-valued logic refers to the *structure* of the domain, and that this implies that the two values are already part *of a domain*.

Günther (2004) goes on to discuss the ontological assumptions of this arrangement. The implication is that everything that exists in the universe is 'monocontextural': it belongs to the universe of being and cannot belong to nothingness. He discusses a range of approaches in philosophy that went beyond the initial monocontextural approach of Aristotle, a good example of which was Hegel. Hegel's recognition that becoming was something that went beyond both being and nothingness implies that contexturalities can overlap with each other and generate a multivalent structure. This last point is worth reiterating. Günther states:

> By showing how Becoming has a component of Being as well as Nihility, he unwittingly laid ground to a theory of 'poly-contexturality'. Because, if we want to establish such a theory, we should not assume that all contexturalities can be linked together in the way a geographical map shows one country bordering on the next in a two-dimensional order. If the contexturality of Becoming overlaps, so to speak, the contexture of Being as well as of Nothingness, and the contexture of Becoming in its turn may be overlapped by a fourth contexture which extends beyond the confines of the first three, we will obtain a multi-levelled structure of extreme logical complexity.
>
> (Günther 2004: 4)

The implication of this for Günther is that the universe is a compound contexture 'composed of an innumerable number of two-valued structural regions' that can run parallel to each other and penetrate each other. One value can belong to two contextures, but its identity changes with respect to each contexture to which it belongs. Although the universe has a strict two-valued structure, this introduces a many-valued structure with respect to identity (Günther 2004). These ideas have been applied in systems theory through the work of Teubner (2000, 2007).

Polycontexturality in systems theory

The idea of polycontexturality has had a significant influence on systems theory. It has enabled Niklas Luhmann to propose a detailed theory of social differentiation but to develop his approach in very particular ways.[3] For Luhmann, systems are divided into different kinds (interactions, organisations and sociey), and societies are in turn divided into systems that perform specific functions, for example, the economy, law, education, medicine and science (Borch 2011). Each function system is monocontextural because it views the world through a singular two-sided code. This singular view cannot be connected with the view of other function systems. Society is therefore composed of fundamentally different 'non-congruent' views on reality (Borch 2011: 90).

Teubner applies these ideas to the problem of the changing status of contracting in society (Teubner 2000, 2007), and his ideas are important enough for us to describe briefly before going on to discuss their relevance to research ethics. Rather than being a simple economic exchange, contracting has become the site of a multiplicity of different 'discursive' projects. This means that a contract can no longer be seen as a unity but rather it is 'fractured into the endless play of discourses. It sounds paradoxical, but one contract is in reality broken up into a multiplicity of contracts' (Teubner 2000: 403). The contract for Teubner (2000) appears to involve three separate projects:

1.   a productive agreement;
2.   an economic transaction;
3.   a legal promise.

Productive agreements can happen within a multiplicity of social worlds; within medicine, distribution, production, science, services, engineering and so on. The contract is always happening under the conditions of a market contract where profit and competition reign supreme. Finally, the contract is a legal project and a time-binding promise that involves rule-producing obligations. These projects are in fact closed to each other, cannot be seen as part of one and the same contract and are all participating in different social dynamics. They are also operatively closed from each other and are heading in different directions (Teubner 2000; 2007).

Teubner (2000; 2007) makes some fundamental observations. He draws on the orthogonal relation between polycontextures embedded within Luhmann's systems theory. Contracts are exposed to contradictory, fractured and very different social rationalities. Indeed, the contract is a 'conflictual relation between colliding discourses, language games, systems, textualities, projects, trajectories' (Teubner 2000: 405). Contracting has to take account of this plurality of discourses as it has dissolved into what Teubner (2000) has termed the multiplicity of different projects existing in different worlds of meaning. The contract, then, exploits the desires and energies of the partners, for the purpose of achieving the contractual end.

This view of contracting moves beyond seeing it as a simple economic exchange; it becomes a 'project'. The purpose of Teubner's (2000) view of the contract is to explore it as an attempt to direct attention away from the obligations of the parties involved towards how the contract constitutes the social system. One contract can put three different discourses into effect. Beneath this is a productive use of the idea of polycontexturality whereby a contract can have several identities running simultaneously in different directions. This brings us to the last point. The contract is also an interdiscursive translation. Put simply, this means that the contract works primarily as a process of mutual translation of discursive projects. In his example, Teubner gave the contract a text that was written in three different languages (legal rights and duties, economic costs and benefits, the project of the work involved and the goods and services). The process of contracting was therefore involved in permanently translating messages from the productive project to the legal project and the economic project.

Embedded within this arrangement is a process of surplus extraction that occurs through a basic *misunderstanding*. In other words, one discourse uses the other in its own terms; it misunderstands the other and creates something new *for itself*. In this sense, then, polycontexturality releases energy and can in fact result in an incredibly productive process. The contract produces a bundle of different rationalities. Not only is it able to very briefly bind these together but it also releases their centrifugal tendencies. The contract, then, sets in motion an ultracyclical movement of different social systems. It makes possible their autopoiesis so that they can make use of each other's cycle of self-reproduction (Teubner 2000).

Applying polycontexturality to the study of research ethics

Luhmann (1995) divides systems into different general types (interactions, organisations and societies). The societies we are most interested in are those that have become differentiated into different functional subsystems. Such societies are polycontextual. We can begin with the assumption that society is composed of multiple systems operating along the lines of their monocontextural distinctions. For us, the most relevant systems are the health system, which operates with the code sick/healthy, the scientific system, which operates with the code true/false, the legal system, which operates with the code legal/not legal, and, finally, the economy, which operates with the code payment/non-payment. Functional subsystems help organise communication along their core monocontextural distinctions. These distinctions are logical in that they involve a sharp and tightly bound distinction between 'what is' and 'what is not'. Not only are these systems cut off from each other but they are also unable to stand outside society in order to describe it. There are, therefore, no priority areas through which to view society and so rather than a hierarchy we have a *heterarchy* (see Chapter 1). There are several claims that result from the concept of polycontexturality. These are as follows:

- There can be no overarching principle, no retreat to a generalisable idea from which to view society.
- All views of society from *all* systems are partial and reflect observers constructions of the world as they see it.
- No one contexture can dominate all others.
- The question of how distinctions used by different contextures are applied, suspended and conditioned by each other is an empirical question of fact for sociology.

In this chapter, the important question is how contextures condition the application of norms in scientific research. In addition, we can also expect to see the same distinction being used by different contextures although we will be sensitive to the fact that when the same distinction is used in different contextures that the meaning will be different. In what follows we have analysed the guidelines produced by the NHS National Research Ethics Service (NRES) which governs all research conducted on patients within the health service in the UK. We have also analysed the guidelines produced by the MRC (2012), which is the primary funding council for medical research in the UK. In contrast to these sources, we have explored the Federation of European Laboratory Animal Science Associations (FELASA) Principles and Practice in Ethical Review of Animal Experiments Across Europe and the Nuffield Council on Bioethics.

Science as a polycontextural project

Each organisation (the NHS, the MRC, FELASA and the Nuffield Council on Bioethics) can be understood as a contexture for ethical communication. How they handle the various distinctions associated with ethics, including the success such distinctions have in conditioning the conduct of science, is the subject of our initial analysis. The first thing worth noting is that most scientific research occurs in the form of a 'project' very much in the manner of Teubner (2000, 2007). Significant proportions of scientific research are therefore conducted as a contract between various different parties.

Each research contract will involve numerous 'discursive' projects and an ultracyclical movement of different social systems. In the same way that any contract can be seen as a productive agreement, an economic transaction and a legal promise, contracted research follows a similar form. Research therefore involves more than simply the scientific system. It can be funded by government or commercial interests, such as pharmaceutical companies, and its outputs will have more than simply a scientific dynamic. Such contracts could be observed in terms of the effects they can have on the ultracyclical movements of the various social systems. But polycontexturality brings with it the potential for conflict and exploitation. It is here that ethics become important.

Dignity, rights and safety: the distinction between subject and object

In the documents we explored, a key form of ethical communication is developed under the principle of dignity. For example, the NHS states that 'research must conform to recognised ethical standards, which includes respecting the dignity, rights, safety and well-being of the people who take part' (Department of Health 2011: section 1.1.1). These concepts direct our attention to the distinction between subjects and objects. Human beings as subjects are not to be treated as objects and (a) should not be harmed in any way, (b) should be treated with respect and (c) are persons who are in possession of rights. Clearly, then, this distinction is an *obvious constraint on the conduct of research*. Research projects that breach these principles will (a) not be funded by the MRC and (b) cannot happen on NHS patients. In this distinction, the subject must always retain its identity as subject.[4]

Yet the distinction is applied in different ways. The subject of NHS ethical communication has dignity and rights whereas the subject of the MRC does not. This difference is important. It indicates the degree to which ethical communication around the distinction is constrained by each organisational contexture. The NHS constructs participants as *individual* subjects who have dignity and rights and by doing so it seeks to enrich the subject status of its subjects. The distinction between subject and object, therefore, can act as both a fundamental constraint and also a positive code which can then be used to promote 'public confidence' in research.

In contrast to the NHS, the MRC makes little or no reference to *the enhancement of participants' well-being* during the research process. The MRC refer to patient 'safety', a concept that is quite distinct from the terms used by the NHS (dignity, rights, safety and well-being). It appears to recognise that while participants have interests (in contrast to rights), these are only recognised at the point at which they may conflict with that of research. In this respect, the goal of the MRC, to enable the production of top-quality research, actually constrains the way in which participants are considered as subjects. Within the MRC document, participants and their qualities are, in fact, often seen as a threat to research (MRC 2012). All of this has to do with personhood and what this means for each contexture.

In this respect, personhood involves a range of different conceptions, and we will return to this topic later in the chapter when we discuss the treatment of animals in research. One such principle is the dignity principle. The research-ethics literature frequently discusses the principle of dignity. Indeed, the concept has been the subject of some considerable criticism (Macklin 2003; Schroeder 2008; Killmister 2010), including some suggestion that it is, in fact, useless (Macklin 2003). In its stronger form, dignity is synonymous with being a subject and is tied to 'upholding personal standards and avoiding humiliation' (Killmister 2010: 160). Such an approach is predicated upon the Kantian understanding of dignity as an inalienable conception inherent in all people, by virtue of them being people. However, the immediate problem with the Kantian definition is that it is transcendental. If dignity is unalienable, it cannot be stripped or threatened through circumstance.

There is, therefore, a debate about the inalienability of dignity (Killmister 2010). This debate, while interesting, examines a norm as a fact. In this respect, the ethical communication measures up the facts of the conduct of research to the norm. The dignity principle seeks to ensure that the subject of research, *as a subject, does not change its status during the research project*. This is interesting for a number of reasons. First, the goal of a project is to move from one state to another, to produce a change of status in something, in this case the truth value of a research question. Second, we know that the research project will be undertaken under the conditions of polycontexturality. As such, the project will have additional effects within numerous different contextures. It will, therefore, be polycontextural in its effects. Finally, the whole point of ethical communication is an act of preservation. *The subject must remain a subject throughout the project*. During the project, researchers have to recognise the potential for their actions to undermine and compromise the subject nature of their participants.

The distinction between subject and object acts to condition ethical communication in scientific research. Depending on the organisational contexture, this distinction is applied differently. It can be used to enhance the status of research subjects as is the case with the MRC's code of ethics. Or it can be used to set boundaries around the kinds of projects that will be funded or not. Finally, we have argued that the distinction between subject and object assigns value to the preservation of subjects as subjects. It therefore enables the status of subjects to be enhanced and protected during the project. But what about instances when human beings participate in research, not in the form of a whole person but in the form of tissue? After all, part of the scandal of Alder Hey in the UK was because of the way the tissue obtained from children was treated. This continues the problem of the subject–object distinction and involves the problem associated with treating human beings as things.

The body in its natural state and the body observed

As we have seen, the distinction between what is and what is not human is a key distinction around which ethical controversies often turn. Human beings (subjects) cannot be treated as 'things' (objects). Treating the human body as a thing can, in fact, violate dignity. This has presented a number of difficulties for scientific research (Looney 1994). One consequence of this distinction, for example, is that human genes cannot be patented. The human body is excluded from being commodified in this way. We are told that 'ownership of the human body is contrary to "ordre public", and that human dignity must be preserved' (Looney 1994: 263). Why is this important? Well, a patent grants a monopoly to a company so that they might be granted the sole right to operate a particular technology for a period of time. This confers obvious advantages to companies that wish to invest in a new area of activity such as the Human Genome Project. Patents and their monopolies encourage investment in advanced science and manufacturing. While the patent system involves enforcing certain rights over intellectual property, these are nonetheless quite limited. This has led to a significant debate when it comes to the human genome. Holding a patent cannot be equated with 'ownership' *but is rather a time-limited and conditional monopoly on the use of an invention or design.* A patent does not give the holder a right to produce, sell or use the object in question but gives the holder a right to stop others from doing so by blocking their use of the technology (Wilkinson 2003).

This has led to an interesting distinction, the distinction between the body in its natural state and the body as it is observed through various technologies. So, while genes are not patentable, they belong to the human body, the 'sequences of nucleotides' which have been obtained through processes of genetic engineering and which have an industrial application, are not excluded from being patentable (Looney 1994: 263). From this perspective, the industrial processes associated with science, the transfer from a state of nature into a state of observation can be patented. This enables the state of nature to become a thing to be observed and then communicated about in science. But it also enables the granting of patents to enable investment in science. The obvious problem is that the distinction between dignity and the body, a real entity, versus the body as an observed entity, cross-cut each other. As a consequence, such distinctions are prone to instability and dispute (Looney 1994). Adopting the perspective of Luhmann (1995) and Günther (2004) enables us to suggest that two distinctions can, in fact, cross-cut each other. Our task should be to explore how these distinctions operate to enable and constrain the contexture of science.

The regulation and practice of DNA patenting comes from two sources: the European Union, in particular the EC Directive on the Legal Protection of Biotechnological Inventions, and secondly, the European Patent Convention and the European Patent Office (EPO). Many see the directive as being mainly concerned with ensuring that the European biotechnology industry is internationally competitive, rather than enforcing ethical constraints through regulation (Wilkinson 2003). The directive does prohibit certain kinds of patenting, and Article 5(1) states, '[t]he human body ... and the simple discovery of one of its elements, including the sequence or partial sequence of a gene, cannot constitute patentable inventions' (Wilkinson 2003: 197). However, the directive does not ban DNA patenting, stating that:

> An element isolated from the human body or otherwise produced by means of a technical process, including the sequence or partial sequence of a gene, may constitute a patentable invention, even if the structure of that element is identical to that of a natural element [for example the body].
>
> (European Parliament and Council Directive 98/44/EC of 6 July 1998 on the Legal Protection of Biotechnological Inventions, 5[2])

As we have already noted, human bodies cannot be treated as 'things'. As a distinction, this clearly acts as an important constraint on scientific communication setting boundaries around the treatment of human beings and their tissue in scientific research. Research that will cause harm to human beings or that treats human tissue as a thing cannot even be considered. However, this distinction can threaten investment in science and has presented particular difficulties for the Human Genome Project. Rather than being suspended or dissolved, the principle of human dignity remains. An alternative distinction is generated between the body in nature and the body in science. In the latter case, the body is *the body as observed*.

In this respect, we can see how different contextures have operated in mutual antagonism to block and then ensure that a very particular scientific project could continue. Initially, the legal system guarded the norm that human beings are not things. In doing so, it observed that any treatment of human tissue as a thing was illegal. Such tissue could not be patented. But the application of the subject–object distinction in this contexture clearly threatened the Human Genome Project in science. In order to enable investment in the Human Genome Project, a new distinction has to be developed: the distinction between the body in nature and the body as observed. The development of this distinction within the legal system subsequently enabled future investment in the project. This enables a commercial body to speculate in a project such as the Human Genome Project while feeling that it can secure future profit. We can see how the contexture of the legal system preserved the original subject–object distinction. This subsequently threatened a whole project in science, and, as a consequence, the legal system had to develop a new distinction (between the body in nature and the body as observed) in order to preserve investment in a science.

The distinction between human and non-human, and harm and benefit in animal experiments

Another area of scientific controversy for at least the past 400 years has been problems associated with conducting experiments on animals (Nuffield Council on Bioethics 2005). Animals possess qualities of sentience, and it has become necessary to evaluate whether or not experiments on them should even be considered appropriate. If we take into consideration the FELASA recommendations, it becomes quite clear that a different set of distinctions apply to experiments on or with animals.

The first point to note is that while animals are recognised as having sentience, they are described as 'non-human'. This is in contrast to the ethical communication on the use of people, where the distinction is between people as subjects and objects. There is a distinction in FELASA and other communications about research ethics and animals between person/non-person and human/non human.

We discussed some of the properties associated with personhood earlier in this chapter, specifically as they relate to dignity, and this has relevance to animals and their treatment generally. It has been suggested that personhood is associated with a range of properties without being precise in defining them (DeGrazia 2006). These include, for example, autonomy, rationality, self-awareness, linguistic competence, sociability, capacity for intentional action and moral agency (DeGrazia 2006: 42). One does not have to have all of these properties to be a person, as demonstrated by non-autonomous people, including children. But a person needs enough of them. As discussed previously, the concept is vague and the boundaries rather arbitrary. The distinction between human and non-human is evident and uncontested in the research-ethics communication about animals as animals are defined as 'non-human'. It is worth noting that this distinction has been challenged. Ryder (2006) has characterised what he terms as the prejudice against non-humans as 'speciesism' and draws a parallel with other forms of discrimination such as racism and sexism. He argues that there is no moral justification between the distinction we impose upon persons and non-persons. Questions of autonomy, rationality, self-awareness and so on are irrelevant, and what matters morally is only that animals experience pain and suffer (Ryder 2006). This, Ryder argues, is sufficient to accord animals similar moral worth in their treatment in scientific research as one would a human participant (Ryder 1975; Singer 2006).

This distinction between human/non-human and seeing animals as non-human overcomes any requirement to discuss the protection of rights and dignity. Therefore, the distinctions of ethical communication in relation to animals are quite distinct from those discussed above involving people. We discover that animal experiments are subject to constant evaluation and ethical justification but this does not involve discussion of animals as 'subjects'. They are not, however, entirely objects. This justification involves considering the possibility that the objectives of the research may well be achieved through other means which may avoid the use of animals. Such evaluations involve exploring to what degree the expertise of those involved in the experiments will ensure the outcomes of the research will be achieved in practice. But fundamental here is that ethical communication about the involvement of animals in research is centred around a harm–benefit calculation (FELASA 2005). The distinction between harm and benefit in relation to the ethics of animal experiments relates to:

> how far the potential, likely and (later) actual benefits of that use can be regarded as 'sufficient' in light of the potential, likely and (later) actual harms that will be caused to the animals ... This ethical weighing is often referred to as a cost-benefit analysis. However, so as avoid inappropriate quantitative or economic implications it is preferable to call the process a harm-benefit assessment.
>
> (FELASA 2005: 13)

This distinction is unstable. Benefits mean different things in different contextures. In relation to the economic contexture, animal experiments entail a cost–benefit evaluation. In relation to scientific communication, they entail a distinction between harm and benefits. On the one hand, the report acknowledges that there is an economic calculation that can be made in relation to animal experiments, but the report seeks to make the calculation a harm–benefit calculation. Can this be interpreted as a distinction for ethical communication in science? We think it can for the following reasons.

The FELASA report was designed to try and bring greater transparency and consistency to European directives on animal experiments. One of its goals was to ensure that:

> Ethical evaluation of scientific projects involving animals should include not only assessment of the harms likely to be, or actually, caused to the animals, and the possibilities for reducing them, but also the quality of the justification for such a use of animals, in terms of the objectives of the project ... and the potential and likely benefits of the work. That is, such ethical evaluation should take the form of a harm-benefit assessment.
>
> (FELASA 2005: 13)

The distinction is clear: that there will be no animal experiments where there can be no direct benefits. The FELASA recommendations seek to bind harm to benefits so that all ethical communication about animal experiments will include such considerations. They also go further to argue for procedures to ensure that this consideration is made throughout scientific projects. If the harm–benefit ratio changes during the experiment, to the point where the harm outweighs the benefits, then the experiment must stop. The distinction is, therefore, a boundary-setting mechanism for scientific experiments that use animals as their subjects.

There are deeper running ethical reasons for this distinction. The avoidance of harm is the stronger side of the distinction, and there is a very good reason for harm to form the primary side of the distinction. It is the basis of all decisions and, simply put, means that all harm should be avoided (Nuffield Council on Bioethics 2005). The application of this side of the distinction to animals contrasts dramatically with its application to human beings. The distinction can be used to justify and at the same time stop experiments on animals. So, on the one hand, by not engaging in research, we may cause harm to human beings and, as such, are breaching the 'do no harm' principle; on the other hand, we should also avoid doing harm to animals, wherever possible. As we can see, this distinction is subject to modification. When it comes to the distinction between animals and humans, there is no mention of dignity or rights for animals, only a weakened distinction of doing no harm *where there is little or no benefit*.

Polyphonic unity and the conditioning effect of organisational purpose

The brief analysis provided in this chapter demonstrates that there are several contextures associated with ethical communication in medical science. When it comes to such communication, it makes sense to consider organisations as 'polyphonic' unities (Åkerstrøm-Andersen 2003). A principal source of polyphonic unity in ethical communication is the purpose of the organisation. The MRC, in its position statement on research ethics, states that it recognises the need for regulation but indicates that a balance needs to be struck between this 'need' and the competing 'need' for 'vital medical research to improve individual and public health' (MRC 2012: 1). Ethical considerations, therefore, should be constrained by the need for research to happen. This contrasts with the NHS Research Ethics Framework in which research is recognised as a core part of the NHS and an important part of improving the health and well-being of the people that the NHS serves (Department of Health 2011: 6). Research in this organisational context is integral to a service whose primary goal is to protect and improve the health and well-being of the population. Polyphonic unity, then, appears to act as a source of constraint to ethical communication within these organisations. On the one hand, it is constrained by the need for research to happen, for example with the MRC, and, on the other, it should be conducted in such a way as not to interfere with the 'care' of the patient.

The unity of each constraint can also have enabling effects for organisations in terms of how they take account of ethics. This appears to involve the recognition of the importance of ethical communications while at the same time preserving the primary goal of the organisation. The NHS has the primary goal of promoting health for the UK population, and this is the unity of its constraint. How does this operate in its communications? The NHS acknowledges that not only is it responsible for the well-being of individuals, it is also responsible for the well-being of the population. By acknowledging this distinction, the NHS can simultaneously communicate about both goals. Research and the generation of knowledge can be seen to enable the achievement of better health for the population and, as such, can ultimately enhance health care in general. In contrast, the primary goal of the MRC is to enable good-quality scientific research (the unity of its constraint) with this primary goal that ethical communications have to be incorporated but with reference to enhancing science rather than acting as a parasitic influence. For the MRC, this is achieved through the language of 'trust'. Often the ethical governance of science has the goal of improving 'public confidence' (MRC 2012: 6). A system based on a lack of trust, it is argued by the MRC, might threaten to produce too much of a burden and may in itself be unethical 'by creating so many barriers that ethical research may be discouraged, even to the point where it may not take place, and this itself may be unethical' (MRC 2012: 6).

Another, more general, constraint on ethical communication appears to be the contexture of science. In the following example, we can see how the NHS expresses the importance of research:

> Research is essential for protecting and improving health and well-being, as well as for achieving modern, effective care services. At the same time, research can sometimes involve an element of risk, because research can involve trying something new. It is important that any risks are minimised and do not compromise the dignity, rights, safety and well-being of the people who take part.
>
> (Department of Health 2011: 8)

In this statement, the promise and essential nature of research is constrained by a consideration of the possible harm that might result. Risks must therefore be 'minimised', but one should *not compromise* dignity (rights, safety and well-being). We would therefore expect NHS research ethics committees to be less tolerant of risks associated with impacts on the dignity (rights, safety and well-being) of participants.

How an organisation sees its environment, or rather the environment of its main activity, also appears to have an impact on the polycontexturalities of research ethics. In this respect, the environment of research can contain objects, animals and human beings, and to these are applied highly nuanced and varied sets of facts and values. What is clear from the Nuffield Foundation on Bioethics and the FELASA document is that the application of the harm–benefit distinction appears to decay depending on the different ways in which facts and values are encountered. It is when we get to the context of the FELASA and the difficulties associated with attempting to review and coordinate the use of animals in science across Europe that we can see how such a broad-reaching organisational context can affect polycontexturality. Here the principal goal or recommendation was the application of a 'tight' distinction between harm and benefit and to apply this distinction throughout European science. In other words, the need to try and provide some guidelines that may or may not be adhered to in future results in the generation of a rigorous distinction between harms and benefit.

Concluding comments

In this chapter we took as our starting point the growth in communication about research ethics and controversies in science either through the misuse of human subjects or human tissue which have resulted in such communication. One consequence of the potential for such controversies appears to have been the generation of ethical reflection. A key question considered both by Luhmann, Haggerty and others is the extent to which transcendental norms can serve as a form of social control. We would like to contribute to this debate further, and alongside the work of Nassehi *et al.* (2008) and Schirmer and Michailakis (2011) the added finding that scientific reflection on ethics involves the use of different distinctions. These include the distinction between the human being as subject and the human being as object, the body in its natural state and the body observed, between harm and benefit and finally between objects, human and non-human animals.

What we have seen is that these distinctions encounter each other but critically they are handled in very different ways according to the contexture in which they are used. For example, we have seen that the human body should not be treated as a thing. It can, however, be observed as an object. Such observation technologies can be patented and controlled as objects. Yet, while the human body should not be treated as an object, the same does not apply to non-human animal bodies. This becomes especially relevant when the distinction of benefit–harm cuts across the body as nature–object distinction. We have discussed the fact that harm is the stronger side of the benefit–harm distinction. Harm should be avoided. Yet, in these communications, it is clear that by not conducting experiments on animals, society can inflict harm on human beings. As a result, it is observed that there can be a demonstrable benefit to inflict harm on animals and the human/non-human distinction, although open to criticism, erodes conflicting moral discourses about causing harm to animals. The strength of avoiding harm remains, however, a weakened moral distinction because there should be no experiment on animals where the harm/benefit distinction is not observed to be beneficial. As a consequence, there is a constant watchfulness on the distinction between harm and benefit throughout scientific projects. It remains an ongoing and constant feature of evaluation during these experiments.

Added to these effects, the contexture of the organisation also has an effect on the use of various distinctions in ethical communication. Interestingly, here the impact of the contexture of the organisation on the application of distinctions associated with research ethics is less predictable and therefore potentially quite revealing. To begin with, the goal of the NHS is to provide health care to individuals and the nation as a whole. As a consequence, it has a very sophisticated view of research ethics involving human subjects. Rather than simply avoiding harm, we find references to dignity, rights, safety and well-being, all of which point to a range of distinctions associated with the subject/object distinction. The MRC's position is less developed. Not only is there less consideration of the range of possible principles for research ethics, the main concern of the statement is, in fact, to ensure that good quality scientific research continues. Yet here the distinction of treating a human being as a subject as opposed to an object remains firmly in place. No harm should be done to a human subject during research projects, their status as subjects should be retained. There is little or no mention of other distinctions.

If we take the FELASA, however, we can see that the contexture of this organisation interacts with the way in which it seeks to reinforce the harm/benefit distinction throughout Europe. It seeks to achieve this without the power to do so. In this respect, we can clearly see that by reinforcing the distinction that ethical communication about animal experiments in Europe would be greatly enhanced. In their review of current practices in Europe associated with the ethics of animal experiments, they discovered that very few countries engaged in reflection on the benefits of such experiments. In other words, by only reflecting on harms, various groups within Europe were not thinking about the benefits that would be gained from an experiment. This is important because by considering benefits this side of the distinction reinforces the principle of doing no harm since if no benefits will accrue then harm should not be done.

Clearly then, when we compare organisational contextures and the distinctions of ethical communication in this way, we begin to see that the manner in which these distinctions are applied within different contextures is of sociological interest. Our analysis confirms the finding of Nassehi *et al.* (2008) that there is certainly an 'interlocking' and a 'recognition of different perspectives'. In addition to this, however, we can also suggest that how each organisational contexture sees the environment of its research has enormous consequences for the application of various distinctions. This is especially the case in the difference between human beings and animals. Each document can be seen as a disintegrated present of distinctions with the goal of enabling research to happen. It does so in a way that clearly takes into account key aspects of the polycontextural environment of research whereby ethical communication can have several paradoxical moral seams running through it simultaneously.

Notes

1   This observer can be the person or an organisation; it can also refer to a particular system such as science or law.

2 The notes taken here are from a reprint of the chapter that was later published online in 2004. All references are to that reprint.
3 See Borch (2011) for a summary.
4 We could push the analysis further and talk about how subjects do, in fact, become objects in science. Such an analysis would no doubt provide us with an interesting example of polycontexturality producing an ultracyclical motion.

References

Åkerstrøm-Andersen, N. (2003) 'Polyphonic Organisations', in T. Bakken and T. Hernes (eds.), *Autopoietic Organization Theory*, Copenhagen: Copenhagen Business School Press.

Borch, C. (2011) *Niklas Luhmann*, London and New York: Routledge.

Degrazia, D. (2006) 'On the Question of Personhood beyond Homo Sapiens', in P. Singer (ed.), *In Defense of Animals*, Oxford: Blackwell, pp. 40–53.

Department of Health (2011) *Governance Arrangements for Research Ethics Committees: A Harmonised Edition*, Leeds: UK Health Departments.

Dingwall, R. (2006) 'Confronting the Anti-Democrats: The Unethical Nature of Ethical Regulation in Social Science', *Medical Sociology Online*, 1: 51–8.

Federation of European Laboratory Animal Science Associations (2005) 'Principles and Practice in Ethical Review of Animal Experiments Across Europe', FELASA Working Group on Ethical Evaluation of Animal Experiments.

Günther, G. (2004) 'Life as Polycontexturality', in G. Günther (ed.), Beiträge zur Grundlegung einer operationsfähigen Dialektik, Band 2, Hamburg: Meiner Verlag, pp. 283–306.

Haggerty, K. (2004) 'Ethics Creep: Governing Social Science Research in the Name of Ethics', *Qualitative Sociology Review*, 27 (4): 391–414.

Killmister, S. (2010) 'Dignity: Not Such a Useless Concept', *Journal of Medical Ethics*, 36: 160–4.

Looney, B. (1994) 'Should Genes Be Patented? The Gene Patenting Controversy: Legal, Ethical, and Policy Foundations of an International Agreement', *Law and Policy International Business*, 26 (1): 231–72.

Luhmann, N. (1995) *Social Systems*, Palo Alto, Calif.: Stanford University Press.

——(2008) 'Are There Still Indispensable Norms in Our Society?' *Soziale Systeme*, 14 (1): 18–37.

Macklin, R. (2003) 'Dignity Is a Useless Concept', *British Medical Journal*, 327: 1419.

Medical Research Council (2012) *Medical Research Council Position Statement on Research Regulation and Ethics*, London: Medical Research Council.

Moeller, H.-G. (2012) *The Radical Luhmann*, New York: Columbia University Press.

Nassehi, A., I. Saake and K. Mayr (2007) 'Healthcare Ethics Committees Without Function? Locations and Forms of Ethical Speech in a "Society of Presents"', in Barbara Katz Rothman, Elizabeth Mitchell Armstrong and Rebecca Tiger (eds.), *Bioethical Issues, Sociological Perspectives* (*Advances in Medical Sociology*, vol. 9), Bingley: Emerald Group Publishing, pp.129–56.

Nuffield Council on Bioethics (2005) *The Ethics of Research Involving Animals*, London: The Nuffield Council.

Panno, J. (2005) *Stem Cell Research: Medical Applications and Ethical Controversy*, New York: Facts on File.

Ryder, R. (1975) *Victims of Science: The Use of Animals in Research*, London: Davis-Poynter.

——(2006) 'Speciesism in the Laboratory', in P. Singer (ed.), *In Defense of Animals*, Oxford: Blackwell, pp. 87–103.

Schirmer, W. and D. Michailakis (2011). 'The Responsibility Principle: Contradictions of Priority-Setting in Swedish Healthcare', *Acta Sociologica*, 54: 267–82.

Schroeder, D. (2008) 'Dignity: Two Riddles and Four Concepts', *Cambridge Quarterly of Healthcare Ethics*, 17: 230–8.

Schuklenk, U. (2000) 'Protecting the Vulnerable: Testing Times for Clinical Research Ethics', *Social Science and Medicine*, 51 (6): 969–77.

Singer, P. E. (2006) *In Defense of Animals*, Oxford: Blackwell.

Teubner, G. (2000) 'Contracting Worlds: The Many Autonomies of Private Law', *Social and Legal Studies*, 9: 399–417.

——(2007) 'In the Blind Spot: The Hybridization of Contracting', *Theoretical Inquiries in Law*, 7: 51–71.

Wald, D. (2004) 'Bureaucracy of Ethics Applications', *British Medical Journal*, 329: 282.

Wilkinson, S. (2003) *Bodies for Sale: Ethics and Exploitation in the Human Body Trade*, London and New York: Routledge.

10 Personal leadership in polyphonic organisations

Morten Knudsen

Two puzzling empirical phenomena form the starting point of this chapter. The first phenomenon is the observation of a huge increase in executive leadership/management degrees and educational programmes paid for by public organisations such as hospitals. In Denmark, for instance, an official governmental goal is for the managers of, for example, hospital departments, schools, kindergartens and elderly homes to have at least a bachelor degree in management before 2015. The second phenomenon is the widespread talk in health care (and other public) organisations about personal leadership. Since the late 1990s, this and related concepts are gaining an ever more prominent and positive position in policy documents, strategy papers and the like. Better leadership is promoted as a general solution to all kinds of problems. In an overview article on leadership in health care, Peck writes:

> First, the current interest in leadership in UK healthcare is relatively recent. Up until the late 1990s the word 'leadership' appeared infrequently in policy pronouncements in healthcare. In contrast, the concept now occupies a prominent position in most major documents issued, for example, by the English Department of Health. In this respect, the UK NHS is merely following a broader trend in the public sector, both nationally and internationally. Storey (2004a) charts the explosion in papers, programmes and projects dedicated to leadership in public services over the preceding ten years.
>
> (Peck 2006)

The initial observations made in the introductory paragraph raise the questions: why the spread of the semantics on personal leadership and why the increasing emphasis on formal management degrees and educational programmes? My thesis is that the focus on leadership education is a reaction to paradoxes in the semantics promoting the importance of personal leadership. The function of degrees and educational programmes is to form the persons at whom the articulated semantics on personal leadership are directed.

Several dynamics play a role in the spread of leadership semantics, not least reforms involving new public management. The policy papers that form part of the empirical basis of this chapter promote leadership as self-evident, the current bet on better leadership viewed as stemming from new insights and a better understanding of the importance of leadership. Leadership studies intensely criticise this self-evidence, for instance, with the use of the term post-heroic leadership (Alvesson and Spicer 2011). This chapter does not concern why the idea of personal leadership might be wrong but rather examines why it has gained such a dominant position. According to Storey, the scientific answer to the question 'Why leadership and why now?' primarily relates to a diagnosis of changes in the competitive environment as 'with high uncertainty, a need for agile and speedy response to customer expectations and client demand – [which] necessitates a shift from the orderly, planned and bureaucratic mode to a more adaptive and entrepreneurial mode' (2004: 20). Storey also mentions isomorphism (or me-tooism, as he calls it), individualisation and changing structures of authority as possible explanations of the spread of leadership ideals.

I suggest a complementary interpretation focusing on changes in the way managers become included in organisations. Inspired in particular by Luhmann's analysis of the relationship between social structure and the ways people can be included in social systems (1989: 149 ff.), I suggest viewing the semantics on personal leadership as a reflection of changes in the social structure of organisations, changes that form new conditions for inclusion or exclusion. My argument is that the current semantics on personal leadership in health-care organisations and other public organisations reflect the polyphony of the organisations. In the polyphonic organisation, the manager finds many roles but no organisationally given unifying position. Instead, 'the person' is introduced as an imagined unity – outside the organisation.

In the following, I demonstrate in more detail how the semantics on personal leadership have developed in a Danish context. Although national variations may exist regarding the timing, the concrete articulations and the problems with which leadership is related, the general trend towards a focus on leadership is not isolated to Denmark. Before turning to the empirical material, I present the central theoretical concepts guiding the interpretation of the material. The theoretical section briefly presents some of the core elements in systems theory's conceptualisation of the relationship between human beings and social systems – under polyphonic conditions.

Inclusion in polyphonic organisations

The relationship between people and society is a classical subject in sociology (as dealt with, for instance, in Durkheim's book on suicide or in Simmel's discussion of how society is possible). Luhmann, however, criticises the use of 'man' or 'human being' as analytical concepts, finding them to be too compact in the sense that there is no operational unity constituting the 'man' (the body, the brain and the consciousness are coupled but they also have their specific reproductions). Instead, he introduces the distinction between psychic and social systems. The theoretical premise is that psychic systems operate based on consciousness, while social systems operate by means of communication (Luhmann 1995: 210 ff.). This sharp division is, on the one hand, a way of raising a productive question, namely, how are social and psychic systems coupled to each other? On the other hand, the sharp division between psychic and social systems is not without a relation to experience: I experience that I cannot say exactly what I think and that there is no causal relationship between communication and consciousness; that I tell you to feel happy does not mean that you actually do feel happy. In addition, psychic and social systems are autopoietic, operationally closed and self-referential. Autopoietic does not mean self-sufficient (for instance, communication cannot exist without the participation of psychic systems). Autopoiesis is a negative concept, i.e. it claims that events (communications) cannot be explained with something behind the events, in other words, the intentions of an actor. That is why systems theory claims that communication communicates. Communication produces itself as communicative elements refer to other elements and get their meaning in this self-referential network.

Keep in mind that social and psychic systems are not identical and cannot exist independently of each other. Structural coupling is the systems theory term for the coupling between operatively closed systems, and it describes the situation in which the complexity of one system is at the disposal of the construction of another system (Luhmann 1989: 162; 2004: 381 ff.). The concept of inclusion denotes one direction in the specific structural coupling between psychic and social systems. Inclusion is a concept for how social systems constituted by communicative operations use psychic systems in their own reproduction. Inclusion is when an autopoietic psychic system operating based on consciousness makes its own complexity available for the construction of social systems (Luhmann 1989: 162). In other words, inclusion stands for communicative strategies for considering human beings as relevant (Nassehi 2007: 111). Inclusion has an effect as it constitutes human beings as persons, i.e. as authors and addresses, in the communication. No one is by nature a legal person, a market player, a researcher, a doctor – only the inclusion by social systems allows people to be such persons.

Various social systems include people differently. Interactions, organisations and function systems have different forms of inclusion. Also, internally between different function systems, the conditions of inclusion and participation differ as the systems, for example, observe with different codes, have different criteria of relevance and use different communicative media. In organisations, people are included in the form of membership roles. According to Luhmann, an organisation is an autopoietic network of recursively connected decisions and communications oriented at decisions

(Luhmann 2000; Seidl and Becker 2005). The organisation draws a boundary to its environment as it decides who is a member and under which conditions. The membership is specified by means of membership roles in the form of expectations concerning who can communicate about what. These expectations form the conditions for how, for example, managers, employees, clients and patients are included in the organisation.

Organisations cannot structure all communication of their members. The communication concerning diagnosis and treatment in the hospital setting, for instance, is especially structured by the medical function system and its programmes. The medical function system is a complex and internally differentiated system with its own code, knowledge and an endless array of often rapidly changing treatment programmes (Luhmann 1983b, 1990; Saake and Vogd 2008; Stollberg 2009). Doctors at hospitals are thus included as members of an organisation (the organisation decides who is allowed to treat which kind of patients), but they are also included in specific function systems. The organisation may try to decide some conditions for how their members are included in the medical function system, but the organisation knows nothing about, for example, oncology, geriatrics or neurology. Here the organisation depends on the inclusion of its members in the medical function system. Likewise, the researcher is a member of a specific university department but is also included in the scientific function system. This double inclusion of both organisation and function system is nothing new. But the diagnosis of polycontexturality and polyphony as presented in the introduction of this book claims that the couplings between organisational and specific function systems have become more contingent. As suggested in the introduction, polyphony is a situation where the distinction in which to frame a decision is undetermined. Is it a medical decision, a financial decision, a legal decision, a political one? Hence, polyphonic conditions potentially comprise multiple inclusion, instead of just double inclusion (Farzin 2012; Højlund 2012).

Polyphony implies that organisational members can be sequentially included in different function systems without a clear hierarchy. Being a medical director who makes medical decisions that also consider the budget, and being a manager in an organisation without a primary code, i.e. being in a situation with uncertainty about whether decisions are primarily medical or financial, are not the same. In the first case, the organisationally decided membership role of the medical director is to be primarily included in the medical function system, while, in the second, the organisation does not decide a membership role in relation to one specific function system.

The assumption is that Danish public organisations have become more polyphonic since around 1980. Financial instruments, quasi-market structures and all kinds of structural reforms have aimed at the creation of autonomous organisations observing themselves as market enterprises. This also means that the structural couplings between specific organisations and specific function systems have a tendency to be replaced by more contingent couplings. The hospital is coupled not only to the medical system but increasingly also to, for example, politics, the mass media and the economic system. These structural changes create new conditions for the inclusion of managers.

This chapter studies these new conditions for inclusion by examining changes in the semantics on the relationship between organisation and manager. The change in semantics is interpreted as a reflection of changes in the conditions of inclusion. I will thus infer backwards from the semantical changes to structural changes. According to systems theory, all actual communication draws on (and reproduces) reservoirs of meaning. Meaning is condensed into concepts, and the semantical apparatus is the available reservoir of meaning and the meaning-processing rules. Semantics refer to generalised available meaning, which is relatively independent of the situation (Luhmann 1980: 19). Concepts such as manager, leadership, employee, quality and health are broad, condensing pools of meaning. Semantics refer to the ways in which social systems describe and understand different phenomena, including themselves. Systems theory distinguishes between structure and semantics and claims that the semantics are not representations but reflections of societal structures. As Luhmann's many historical analyses of semantical changes demonstrate, semantics are neither independent nor direct representations of structural changes (1980). The relations call for an interpretation. A further characteristic of semantics is that they do not follow the boundaries of individual organisations. In the public sector, we can observe organisations that have developed new semantics as one of their main performances. Organisations such as Local Government Denmark, the Ministry of Finance and the State Employer's Authority produce semantics facilitating the (self-)interpretations of the many individual organisations.

Changing semantics on the organisation–manager relationship

Based on the assumption of changing conditions of inclusion following polyphony, this section describes how the changes in inclusion are reflected in the semantics on the relationship between organisation and managers. The empirical material analysed consists of approximately sixty documents dating from 1945 to 2010, though the majority are from 1980–2010. The criteria for inclusion was that the document had to relate to management development/education in the Danish public sector, a topic chosen initially due to the growing focus on management development/education. Working with the documents made it clear that the perceived need for education had to do with changes in the relationship between organisation and manager. Relevant databases at public libraries and research libraries have been used. In addition to using the section on historical sources in Rennison's (2007; 2011) research on the genealogy of management, direct contact with key individuals associated with leadership development in health care made it possible to identify as many relevant documents as possible. The documents collected were reviewed in order to identify two variables: (1) the relationship between organisation/manager; and (2) the relationship between manager/person.

The organisation–manager relationship

The emergence of personal-leadership semantics is closely related to changes in the way the relationship between organisation and manager is articulated. Material from the 1980s and 1990s places an increasing emphasis on management, which is ascribed a crucial role in the attempt to make the public sector ever more efficient. The notion of leadership becomes more prominent and is combined with terms such as 'strong and visible management' (Finansministeriet 1990: 2). The term 'managerial capacity' is also introduced. In 2001, the Ministry of Finance asserts that 'management is the key to the development of the public sector ... management is among the most essential preconditions for an efficient public sector' (Finansministeriet 2001: 1).[1] This emphasis on management is part of an inversion of the relationship between organisation and manager. A 1994 government report claims that the role of the manager is changing rapidly. While the role of the manager is to steer, control and report to superiors, leadership means deciding about and communicating goals in order to inform, involve and motivate employees (Finansministeriet 1994: 165). The manager is thus much more important in the constitution of the organisation. Instead of being given roles, the manager must determine the goals of the organisation. In other words, motivation is not given but must be created by the manager. In another example, the Ministry of Finance states: 'They [the managers] must be able to lay down general targets for the organisation, which are then translated into concrete work plans. They must secure that the organisation is ready to deviate from the plans if it becomes necessary' (Finansministeriet 1990: 4). Not only should managers decide about goals and plans, but they should also ensure that the organisation can deviate from the plans.

Local Government Denmark discusses whether holding management responsible for the results of an entire organisation is fair. The answer is 'yes' as, '[t]he manager does have a crucial influence on the organisation ... The manager is very much indeed responsible for the production of the *preconditions* that allow the organisation to achieve its results, e.g., by means of personnel management, development and a holistic view' (Kommunernes landsforening 2001: 8).

The idea is not that a bureaucratic structure assigns the roles, tasks and functions of the manager, but rather the opposite. The organisation is given by the manager, who is made responsible for creating the preconditions for organisational production. Or, as a 1990 Ministry of Finance report states, '[t]he managers should be able to see their own organisation from the outside and constantly adjust its services to the change of needs and expectations in the environment' (Finansministeriet 1990: 3). Similar ideas exist in other documents. A State Employer's Authority report states, for instance, that '[g] ood management in development is a precondition for the performance of tasks and the continuous development of the workplaces of the state now and in the future' (Personalestyrelsen/Finansministeriet 2003: 16).

The idea that managers come before the organisation they have a responsibility for constituting raises the question as to which position this is done from. If the manager constitutes the organisation, what, then, constitutes the manager? The semantics concerning personal leadership is an answer to this question.

The manager–person relationship

As mentioned above, the semantics analysed demonstrate that an inversion of the organisation–management relationship has occurred and that the manager is increasingly articulated as the one who constitutes the organisation and not the other way round. The semantics show how the inversion of the organisation–manager relationship caused an increasing interest in 'the person'.

From around 1980, we see a growth in the attempts to define good management and good leadership. This attempt goes hand in hand with the recognised focus on management. The prevailing logic was that management is what is needed and therefore good management must be defined. In the 1980s, this is typically framed as a discussion of management roles, while in the 1990s there is an increasing focus on the person. Management is seen as something constituting the organisation, which means the manager cannot (only) be seen as an organisationally defined role with formal competencies, duties and limitations. The organisation defines the role while the person and personal leadership are articulated as something extra-organisational. This raises the question of upon what grounds does the manager operate if not on organisational ones. Here it is claimed that 'the individual's opportunities for preoccupation/introspection and development become the platform for the manager' (Kommunernes Landsforening 1997: 53). The platform is no longer the formal position in the organisation but the individual's opportunities for preoccupation.

Today, good management is understood to mean that the manager is 'accepted and respected as the natural leader' (*Overenskomstforeningen og Foreningen af Tjenestemænd og Chefer i DJØF* 1995: 6). Instead of the organisational manager, we now have the natural leader or personal leader:

It is required that the manager contributes with the personal leadership, that the manager has a personal vision and that the manager can create a collective vision. The only opportunity you have as a manager for

creating space for your own behavior is by making your own position clear. This is where the benefit should be from the personal leadership.
(Kommunernes Landsforening 1997: 53)

By the end of the 1990s, the untranslated English word 'leadership' is introduced into the discussion. For instance, a Local Government Denmark text states that: *'lederen skal også udøve* "leadership"' (Kommunernes Landsforening 2000: 6), which translates as the manager should also practise leadership. The English word 'leadership' is introduced and used as if it were a well-known concept, which it was not in a Danish context at that time. Ideas concerning vision, courage and motivation are typical in the description of personal leadership, for example: 'they should be engaged in maintaining their personal motivation in the job' (Kommunernes Landsforening 2000: 30); '[m]anagement is carried by personality and presupposes personal leadership' (Finansministeriet 2001: 39); and 'good management presupposes personal leadership, where the personal integrity of the manager, the ability to inspire and fill with enthusiasm and responsibility are important elements' (Erhvervsministeriet/Finansministeriet 2001: 3). And more unfolded:

The Government believes that brave and visionary management is one key to a common exploitation of the possibilities of the knowledge society. Management that has the will and the courage to move the frontiers for what we thought possible and which dares to challenge old habits, values, and ideas.
(Erhvervsministeriet/Finansministeriet 2001: 1)

Management is *no longer* related to values such as conscientious, carefulness and correctness but to values such as audacity, determination and farsightedness, as the following quote illustrates:

Good public management is very much about will, courage and visions. It is a misunderstanding to confuse management with rules and funding. Management is based on attitudes and values and this is why management plays a pivotal role for the culture at the workplace. The management is the driving force in the creation of a culture in which learning and development is in the centre. Where changes are seen as challenges instead of threats, and where everybody is concerned about contributing to the whole.
(Erhvervsministeriet/Finansministeriet 2001: 8)

First, there is a distinction between rules and attitudes/values. The latter is related to the managers as persons (their will, courage and visions). Second, there is the idea of management as a driving force behind the constant changes in an organisation. Management should be personal, and a central aspect of personal leadership is that it must be a driving force in making constant changes. Previously, the manager was manager as he was included as a member in an organisation. With the emergence of the semantics on personal leadership, however, this understanding is supplemented with the opposite idea, i.e. that the manager is constituted outside of the organisation.

The focus on the person also becomes mirrored in formal management degrees and educational programmes. The State Employer's Authority describes the new Master in Public Governance as follows: '[p]ersonal and social competencies play an important role in all management functions. Therefore the development of the participant's personal leadership is an integrated part of the master degree' (Personalestyrelsen 2009: 2). The personal element is institutionalised as part of the formal management degree or educational programmes and is thus, paradoxically, not only up to the individual manager to define.

The semantics on personal leadership is an attempt to articulate a kind of unity partly outside the organisation. The result is that managers become managers by means of their personality. It is nothing new that organisations deal with persons. Organisations constantly contend with both roles and persons. As Elena Esposito states,

> [i]n modern society organizations bring into practice the sociological distinction of person and role, where the person stands for individual singularity and the role for social reliability: Exactly because of this, organizations have become indispensable and have spread more and more. But because of this there are also problems: the difficult constellation of unpredictability and planning, of creativity and control, emerges in classical issues such as the distinction of formal and informal organization, or of hierarchical power and authority. The problem is always to recognize and use the person under the role, without letting in the uncontrollable variety of individuals.
>
> (2011: 609)

Everyone is unique and unpredictable as an individual but not as members of an organisation. Membership is a question of role. Consequently, personal leadership is a paradoxical membership and represents the re-entry of the person in the role, which is to be personal and which translates into inclusion also being a question of self-enrolment (Andersen 2013: 38 ff.). The call for personal leadership then becomes a call for organisationally unprogrammed inputs to the organisational communication. This type of membership also represents an opening for more variance or innovation in the organisation as the contradictory call to the leader now becomes, 'We expect you to be unpredictable.' In this perspective, the emergence of the semantics on personal leadership expresses a change towards more unpredictability and less control based on current ideals of change and innovation, which are exceedingly explicit in the semantics.

But is the ideal of change and the related call for person-based variation a full explanation for the semantical changes described and for the increasing emphasis on management education? Several dynamics are presumably in play simultaneously. In the following, I suggest a complementary interpretation based on the identification of organisational polyphony and expound on the two characteristics described in the brief analysis above: (1) that management increasingly is seen as having a position outside the organisation that involves the power to, for example, constitute, transform and develop the organisation; and (2) that this outside is viewed as the personality of the manager. The changes in semantics are then interpreted in relationship to the increasing organisational polyphony identified.

Personal leadership semantics as a reflection of polyphonic inclusion

The described semantical changes can be related to different rationalities. In the policy documents studied, the changes are often coupled to an ideal of change and innovation as the managers are ascribed the role of mover, of change agent, of incorporating the force that can drive the organisation forward. In the scientific literature, the emergence of the personalising semantics has mainly been interpreted in two different ways. First, it has been interpreted as the increasing amount of insight into the importance of the human factor, an idea that traces its origins from the Hawthorne experiments to the human-resources thinking currently peaking in the discourses on authentic leadership (Gardner *et al.* 2005), appreciative inquiry (Cooperrider and Whitney 2005) and emotional intelligence (Goleman 1995). These researchers emphasise the importance of the *person* as an important but also extra-organisational factor in organisational life. This humanistic interpretation has been criticised by authors who interpret the interest in the person as a part of neoliberal forms of steering and control. Thus, the second way is reflected in the work of authors such as Dean (2007) and Miller and Rose (2008), who discuss personalisation as part of a new type of neoliberal government. Persons are made responsible for their own health and fortune. Especially inspired by Foucault, these studies look at various technologies of the self, focusing on power, knowledge and subjectivity relations – and the technologies supporting and creating the self-governing subjects. These technologies are then related to governance, and the self is seen as part of the governance. According to this literature, one primary social dynamic exists: the will to govern. As Maasen and Sutter write:

> From this perspective, all practices concerned with (self-)education, (self-) management, (self-)therapy, or counseling can be regarded as pivotal governmental techniques in that they perfectly coalesce technologies of domination (e.g., the wish to educate) and technologies of self (e.g., the wish to become educated).
>
> (2007: 9)

Systems theory would not contest that the focus on self, subjectivity and personality can be related to increasing insight or the emergence of still more subtle governmental techniques. Systems theory can offer, however, a supplementary explanation based on its theoretical conception of the relationship between social structures and how individuals are included in social systems.

The interpretation below is inspired by Luhmann's analysis of the relationship between social structure (differentiation), inclusion and semantics (1989: 149 ff.). He argues that the semantics emerging in the eighteenth century on individuality are a reaction to the structural changes in society concerning the conditions for inclusion (Luhmann 1989: 162). From the sixteenth century, society changed from being based primarily on stratificatory differentiation to being based on functional differentiation. People in a functionally differentiated society, instead of being represented as a person in just one system, take part in several function systems (religion, the economy, law, politics); they are no longer offered a societal position as a whole (Nassehi 2007: 112). But if the person is only partially included in different societal systems what then is the individual as a unit? The inherent risk of multi-inclusion is the absence of clear expectations and predictability, i.e. of too much openness and uncertainty regarding the possible behaviour of both oneself and of others. The response to this risk becomes individualisation. The human being must be individualised and must find and declare an identity 'so his behaviour in this only for him relevant constellation can again *be made expectable for others according to his individual person*' (Luhmann 2008: 126, own translation). The semantics on individuality make it possible to imagine that the person as a unity is constituted outside society, as something unknown (black box, spontaneous). Individuality is a place imagined outside social systems, and the individual becomes the adress for the totality of different societal expectations. The semantics on individuality (including, for example, individual human rights and individual freedom) do not mean that individual human beings become more independent of society. The semantics of individuality can even have a compensatory function for stronger dependencies (Luhmann 1989: 160).

My suggestion is to make a similar interpretation of the personal-leadership semantics emerging today in relation to public organisations. The individual doctor or nurse, for example, may, to a larger degree, stick to one function system. But managers are typically included in different streams of communication related to different function systems. In the semantics on public organisations, we see a growth in the management roles described. They become more and more complex, the list of characteristics growing ever longer. The Danish Ministry of Finance, for instance, states, 'the management role in the public sector has been changing rapidly in recent years. Previously, the first priority of the management role was the professional content, and the method of working was primarily a question of control. Today there is a demand for a much more complex management role' (Finansministeriet 1994: 165). This complex management role can be viewed as a consequence of organisational polyphony and the multi-inclusion of the managers in different function systems. The multi-inclusion in many roles raises the issue of what *the* manager is; what unifies the various roles? Without a centre that unites the different function systems, the response becomes to construct the unit of the manager outside the organisation, i.e. in the person. The above analysis illustrates how the organisation–manager relationship became reversed, the manager now expected to constitute the organisation from a position on the outside. This position is increasingly identified with personal leadership. The manager has been moved out of the organisation and becomes a manager specifically by being on the outside, i.e. by exclusion.

The emphasis of the personal leadership can thus be interpreted as a semantic construction that makes it possible to imagine a unity across many roles. The construction of this unity outside the organisation is paradoxical as it exists particularly within the organisational semantics and in so far *inside* the organisational communication about an outside. The construction of personal leadership in polyphonic organisations is parallel to the construction of the individual as a reflection of new conditions of inclusion in the functionally differentiated society. In both situations, the partial inclusion in different function systems brings up the issue of the unity of the person. And in each case, the unity in question becomes an outer social unity. Both the individual and the manager can no longer be defined by means of inclusion but only by exclusion. The semantics on personal leadership reflect the problem of inclusion under polyphonic conditions but end up presenting the symptom of the problem, namely the exclusion of the managers as a positive goal. Instead of dealing with the problem of inclusion under polyphonic conditions, the semantics reproduce classical notions of the heroic, outstanding and natural leader.

One of the various impacts of the semantics on personal leadership is that they create new expectations concerning managers and a need to identify the outside position, the person, more precisely. This produces an organisational dilemma. On the one hand, it generates an enormous interest in the person, while on the other, the person is constructed as the outside of the organisation. In addition, personal leadership is celebrated but raises the question of whether the person can be brought back in and made socially addressable. The next section argues that education is one way of dealing with this dilemma.

Education as compensation

Let me begin with a few empirical facts. Before 1980, Danish policy documents on matters such as qualifications and education did not put much emphasis on the manager as an individual person, generally focusing on personnel instead. This started to change in the 1980s and 1990s, culminating in the 2000s with a dramatic increase in management education. Today, an official governmental goal is for all the heads of organisations such as kindergartens, elderly care homes and schools to have at least a bachelor degree in management before 2015. Within the framework of the 2007 quality reform, representatives from all three levels of government (Government, Local Government Denmark and Danish Regions) decided that all public managers should have the right to earn a degree in management. Since 2007, many management/leadership programmes at the bachelor and graduate level have been developed. In 2007, around seventy-five public managers were enrolled in the executive master's programme at Copenhagen Business School (CBS). Today, there are more than 700 public managers in master's programmes at CBS, approximately 30 per cent of whom work in healthcare-related organisations, primarily hospitals. Also many in-house programmes have been developed recently. For instance, the Capital Region of Denmark, one of five Danish hospital owners, has developed a large in-house leadership-development programme that all of its leaders (more than 2,500, mainly from the hospitals) are required to attend.

Older governmental reports warn against participation in too many courses and educational activities because they are perceived as taking time away from the real tasks at hand, indicating that it is not a law of nature that leadership development should take form as formal education. Traditionally, Danish managers have become managers based on a combination of recruitment and learning by doing. Other ways of improving leadership skills besides postgraduate education include job rotation, mentoring and experience-exchange groups. Despite this, the focus on formal education today is enormous, which is the reason it makes sense to discuss not only *why* we see this huge investment in leadership development but also why it takes the *form* of formal education. I propose that this strong focus relates to a dilemma inherent to the semantics on personal leadership, an idea that will be further elaborated upon in the next section.

Education and the dilemma between the organised manager and the capricious manager

Above we saw how polyphony creates new conditions for inclusion and how this is reflected in the semantics focusing on personal leadership. According to the semantics, organisations depend on individuals who are ascribed a position outside the organisation. This raises the matter of how the organisation can avoid the arbitrariness of managers. The personalisation of management is viewed as the way to go, but concessions are made because not all leaders are professional or qualified enough to live up to what is expected of them. A natural leader is desirable, not an unorganised leader. The question is how organisations can equip managers to meet expectations without losing the sought-out traits of a manager on the outside. Educating managers and providing them with additional qualifications runs the risk of programming, domesticating and organising them, i.e. of suffocating the function the leaders are ascribed from their position outside the organisation that allows them to move the organisation. The manager is articulated as a force that comes before the organisation and that constitutes the organisation, which means that it becomes problematic for the organisation to design the programmes that develop the leader. The question becomes how organisations can build personal leadership without structuring and thus destroying it.

This dilemma generates an organisational interest in the processes in which the self and the personality of the managers are created. Reflection (self-reflection, self-management, reflexive practitioners) has been one of the responses to the dilemma described. The logic is simple: if managers are no longer (fully) constituted by the organisation, they must constitute themselves via self-reflection. Creating reflective managers (see, for instance Adriansen and Knudsen 2013, Ahmad *et al.* 2013; Gray 2007; Hibbert 2013) and reflective practitioners (Schön 1983) has become a widespread goal. The idea is that as the unit of the manager is excluded from the organisation, managers must become self-reflexive in order to stabilise the self outside of the organisation. Reflexivity is a stabilising mechanism that makes having certain expectations possible.

Reflexivity can produce, however, contingency just as well as stability. As Luhmann states, 'you cannot in yourself find the substance, you need in order to define yourself' (2008: 127, my translation). There is a risk that the self does not find much when it starts to reflect or that it dissolves what is found. As a result, calling for reflexivity alone is insufficient. The need also exists to influence the reflective self-constituting processes of the managers. An interest in education emerges. My argument is that leadership degrees and educational programmes have emerged as an attempt to compensate for the risks involved in the semantics privileging the manager above the organisation. The theoretical distinction between education and socialisation can enlighten this argument.

While inclusion is a concept concerning how social systems let psychic systems become relevant, the concept of socialisation denotes the other direction in the coupling between psychic and social systems. Socialisation means that psychic systems use communication (meaningful goals, concepts, figures, metaphors, sentences) to structure and inform the processes of consciousness (Luhmann 1987: 163). Luhmann suggested that education is related to socialisation and defined it as an arrangement of social systems specialised to change persons and speed socialisation (1987: 182 ff; 2002: 48 ff.). Education is the communicative activity in itself, while socialisation is always self-socialisation as psychic systems are operatively closed. Communication is communication, and, because of the operative closure, there is no causality in how it influences the psychic system (as there is no causality in how psychic systems influence communication processes). Socialisation is not a question of the simple transfer of meaning or of patterns of conformity. Psychic systems can accept or reject the offered meaning.

The distinction between education (as communication) and socialisation (as the activity of psychic systems) and the operative closure of psychic systems points out the improbability of education. Why should the consciousness structure itself and give itself the content that the communication wants it to have? Education is communication directed towards the change of psychic systems, but because of the operative closure of psychic systems it is the psychic systems themselves that decide the effects of the educational activities. Educational communication can be rejected, ignored or transformed. The communication cannot control its own effects in the socialisation of the psychic systems that it is directed towards. Psychic systems can, based on their operative closure, pursue conformity or rejection. For instance, Luhmann points out that there are greater opportunities for individualisation in rejection than in conformity (many parents will recognise this) (1987: 186).

Turning back to the empirical material shows that the increase of *formalised* management degrees and education programs are an answer to two issues, namely, (1) how to educate without defining the content of the communication (in relation to the dilemma between the organised and the capricious manager); and (2) the improbable acceptance of education, which will be explored further below.

How to educate without defining the content of the communication

We can interpret the use of formal degrees and education programmes as a way to avoid defining the content of the education. If the manager is observed as an external force, the energiser that can constitute the organisation from the outside, then it becomes ambivalent for the organisation to be too precise in formulating the form and content of management degrees or educational programmes. One response to this issue is that organisations can let others define the content of the educations, for example, consultancy companies that design leadership-development programmes in (and with) larger organisations, or educational organisations that design and offer management degrees or education programmes. The use of formal educations can be seen as a system displacement of the dilemma between unprofessional leaders (i.e. the risk of arbitrariness) and domestication (i.e. the risk of habitual instead of innovative leaders). The task of qualifying and speeding the self-socialisation of leaders is displaced by education as a functional system and by educational organisations. Thus the organisations of the managers relieve themselves of the task of deciding the make-up of the leaders' qualifications. The result is that we have thousands of public managers earning degrees or attending educational programmes in which the teachers typically have a rather superficial knowledge about the tasks and organisations of the leaders or students, which is what they are in an educational setting. These teachers nonetheless develop the form and content of the educational programmes.

The improbable acceptance of education

As organisations, hospitals decide certain values, goals, strategies, management platforms and codes of good governance. Even though they communicate about these areas and perhaps have even attended courses on values, it does not mean that the managers and the employees identify themselves with the values. Instead, they may ignore them, forget them or find them ridiculous, hypocritical, meaningless. Critical questions should perhaps be posed, such as, 'Would you trust someone who actually took such organisational communication seriously? Would it not be regarded as a lack of self-dependence?' It is not easy for organisations to succeed in educating managers. As a result, the introduction of formal degrees and education programmes can be seen as a way to increase the probability of educational acceptance, and they can be seen as social support measures that can neutralise the probability of educational failure. There is, for instance, less resistance if you have to pay for the education (with money or time). Or if a scientific institution is in charge of the educational programme rather than the organisation itself. Moreover, if a widely recognised diploma is awarded, there is less resistance than if one's efforts only count in a single specific organisation.

Education as a functional system has its own codes and programmes. What it contributes and the difference it makes in the organisations from which managers come are of less relevance to the educational system, which also has difficulties in observing and controlling its effects outside its own boundaries. This, on the other hand, also means that public organisations can arrange themselves so they do not have to take management-school concepts and theories too seriously (which is a frustrating situation many newly graduated managers experience). Instead, public organisations can continue to be based on the socialisation of the managers in their daily interactions.

Final discussion

This chapter argues that the semantics of personal leadership reflect changing conditions of inclusion in the polyphonic organisation. The semantics of personal leadership reflect a structural problem concerning inclusion. Instead of reflecting on it as a problem, however, the semantics claim that personal leadership (i.e. the excluded manager) is a solution to all kinds of problems.

Polyphony means organisational complexity. The semantics on personal leadership reduce this complexity by introducing a definition of the leader as someone who is expected to constitute (energise, motivate, direct) the organisation from the outside. This, in turn, creates a need to change the managers in ways so that their decisions are not based on arbitrary ideas and impulses. In other words, this creates a need to help the empirical managers live up to the expectations in the semantic.

The current interest in management degrees and educational programmes is a reaction to the fact that the semantics construct a fiction about the person, which then raises the issue of how to make this fiction real. Public-sector organisations can claim that they have responsibly upgraded the qualifications of managers by providing them with educational opportunities. The educational system can (as an autopoietic, operatively closed communication system) do what it does: teach managers to be students (to read papers, to carry out academic analyses, do assignments). A basic question nonetheless remains in this hazy process that displaces the task of education to the educational system: how is the definition of a polycontexturally competent managers and how can they be supported?

This situation begs the question as to what competencies the managers/students should acquire, and what influence do the degrees and educational programmes have on managers' decisions? The empirical material examined in this study does not provide a sufficient evidence to address this question. One hypothesis, however, is that the professionalisation of management by means of education means that, for example, generalised notions of organisations and steering (i.e. the theoretical knowledge of management textbooks), mediated by the managers, become a more important context for organisational decision-making. It is ironic that the semantic reflection of polyphony risks leading to a management education that, by means of textbook learning, produces generic, simplified descriptions of the organisation. The managers do not necessarily learn to be autonomous and able to cope with contingency. They may instead be trivialised in the sense that they get certain concepts of what organisations and management are or should be. Both the semantics and the educations run the risk of reproducing notions of the heroic leader as someone who constitutes the organisation. Personal-leadership semantics and educational programmes may be self-fulfilling prophecies, with the semantics having an organising effect and influencing the structure of organisations. Hospitals may structure themselves to give managers more influence, and managers may begin starting to believe that they really do constitute the organisation. This may result in organisations that end up making themselves more and more inferior compared to their own polyphonic complexity.

Notes

1 The quotes are translated by the author. In Danish there is no distinction made between management and leadership – there is just one word: *ledelse*. This poses problems in the translation of quotes. I have chosen to translate *leder* and *ledelse* to 'manager' and 'management', respectively, as they are the most generic terms. In recent years we have witnessed the emergence of the terms *lederskab* and *det personlige lederskab*, which is a direct translation from the English terms 'leadership' and 'personal leadership'. As a result, I translate *lederskab* as 'leadership' and *det personlige lederskab* as 'personal leadership'.

References

Adriansen, H. K and H. Knudsen (2013) 'Two Ways to Support Reflexivity: Teaching Managers to Fulfil an Undefined Role', *Teaching Public Administration*, 31 (1): 108–23.

Ahmad, Y., J. C. R. Nielsen, J. Raine and M. Synnot (2013) 'Editorial: Special Issue on Developing the Reflexive Public Manager', *Teaching Public Administration*, 31 (1): 3–5.

Alvesson, M. and A. Spicer (eds.) (2011) *Metaphors We Lead By: Understanding Leadership in the Real World*, London and New York: Routledge.

Andersen, N. Å. (2013) *Managing Intensity and Play at Work: Transient Relationships*, Cheltenham: Edward Elgar.

Cooperrider, D. L. and D. Whitney (2005) *Appreciative Inquiry: A Positive Revolution in Change*, San Francisco, Calif.: Berrett-Koehler.

Dean, M. (2007) *Governing Societies, Political Perspectives on Domestic and International Rule*, New York: Open University Press.

Durkheim, E. (2002) *Suicide: Studies in Sociology*, London and New York: Routledge.

Esposito, E. (2011) 'Originality through Imitation: The Rationality of Fashion', *Organization Studies*, 32 (5): 603–13.

Farzin, S. (2012) 'Inklusion/Exklusion', in O. Jahraus, A. Nassehi, M. Grizelj, I. Saake, C. Kirchmeier and J. Müller (eds.), *Luhmann Handbuch: Leben-Werk-Wirkung*, Stuttgart: J. B. Metzler, pp. 87–8.

Gardner, W. L., B. J. Avolio and F. O. Walumbwa (2005) *Authentic Leadership Theory and Practice, Origins, Effects and Development*, Amsterdam: Elsevier Science.

Goleman, D. (1995) *Emotional Intelligence*, New York: Bantam Books.

Gray, D. E. (2007) 'Facilitating Management Learning: Developing Critical Reflection through Reflective Tools', *Management Learning*, 38 (5): 495–517.

Hibbert, P. (2013) 'Approaching Reflexivity through Reflection: Issues for Critical Management Education', *Journal of Management Education*, 37 (6): 803–27.

Højlund, H. (2012) 'Hybrid Inclusion: Multiple Inclusion Mechanisms in the Modernized Organisation of Danish Welfare Services', in N. T. Thygesen (ed.), *The Illusion of Management Control: A Systems Theoretical Approach to Managerial Technologies*, Basingstoke: Palgrave Macmillan, pp. 87–107.

Luhmann, N. (1980) *Gesellschaftsstruktur und Semantik, Bd. 1*, Frankfurt: Suhrkamp.

——(1983b) 'Medizin und Gesellschaftstheorie', *Medizin, Mensch, Gesellschaft*, 8 (3): 168–75.

——(1987) *Soziologische Aufklärung 4: Beiträge zur funktionalen Differenzierung der Gesellschaft*, Opladen: Westdeutscher Verlag.

——(1989) *Gesellschaftsstruktur und Semantik, Bd. 3*, Frankfurt: Suhrkamp.

——(1990) 'Der medizinische Code', *Soziologische Aufklärung*, vol. 5, Frankfurt: Suhrkamp, pp. 176–88.

——(1992) 'Die Universität als organisierte Institution', *Universität als Milieu*, Bielefeld: Haux, pp. 90–9.

——(1995) *Social Systems*, Palo Alto, Calif.: Stanford University Press.

——(2000) *Organisation und Entscheidung*, Opladen: Westdeutscher Verlag.

——(2002) *Das Erziehungssystem der Gesellschaft*, Frankfurt: Suhrkamp.

——(2004) *Law as a Social System*, Oxford: Oxford University Press.

——(2008) *Soziologische Aufklärung 6: Die Soziologie und der Mensch*, Wiesbaden: VS Verlag für Sozialwissenschaften.

Maasen, S. and B. Sutter (eds.) (2007) *On Willing Selves: Neoliberal Politics vis-à-vis the Neuroscientific Challenge: Neoliberal Politics and the Challenge of Neuroscience*, Basingstoke: Palgrave Macmillan.

Miller, P. and N. Rose (2008) *Governing the Present: Administering Economic, Social and Personal Life*, Cambridge: Polity.

Nassehi, A. (2007) 'The Person as an Effect of Communication', in S. Maasen and B. Sutter (eds.), *On Willing Selves: Neoliberal Politics vis-à-vis the Neuroscientific Challenge: Neoliberal Politics and the Challenge of Neuroscience*, Basingstoke: Palgrave, pp. 100–20.

Peck, E. (2006) 'Leadership and Its Development in Healthcare', in K. Walshe and J. Smith (eds.), *Healthcare Management*, Maidenhead: Open University Press.

Rennison, B. W. (2007) 'Historical Discourses of Public Management in Denmark: Past Emergence and Present Challenge', *Management and Organizational History*, 2 (5): 5–26.

——(2011) *Ledelsens genealogi: Offentlig ledelse fra tabu til trend*, Copenhagen: Samfundslitteratur.

Saake, I. and W. Vogd (eds.) (2008) *Moderne Mythen der Medizin: Studien zur organisierten Krankenbehandlung*, Wiesbaden: VS Verlag für Sozialwissenschaften.

Schön, D. (1983) *The Reflective Practitioner: How Professionals Think in Action*, London: Temple Smith.

Seidl, D. and K. H. Becker (eds.) (2005) *Niklas Luhmann and Organisation Studies*, Copenhagen: Liber and CBS Press.

Simmel, G. (1992) Soziologie: Untersuchungen über die Formen der Vergesellschaftung, Frankfurt: Suhrkamp.

Stollberg, G. 2009 'Das medizinische System: Überlegungen zu einem von der Soziologie vernachlässigten Funktionssystem', *Soziale Systeme*, 15 (1): 189–217.

Storey, J. (2004) (ed.) *Leadership in Organizations: Current Issues and Key Trends*, London: Taylor & Francis.

Empirical documents refered to in the chapter

Erhvervsministeriet/Finansministeriet [Ministry of Business and Growth/Ministry of Finance] (2001) *Regeringens ledelsespolitiske redegørelse.*

Finansministeriet [Ministry of Finance] (1990) *Statens lederpolitik i 90'erne.* Finansministeriet[Ministry of Finance], Administrations- og Personaledepartementet [Administration and Personnel Department].

——(1994) *Medarbejder i staten – ansvar og udvikling.*

——(2001) *Ledelse på dagsordenen.*

Overenskomstforeningen og Foreningen af Tjenestemænd og Chefer i DJØF (1995) *Lederudvikling i den offentlige sektor. Rapport fra en arbejdsgruppe om lederudvikling.*

Kommunernes Landsforening [Local Government Denmark] (1997) *Alle regnbuens farver. Udvikling i kommunal topledelse.* Copenhagen: Forlaget Kommuneinformation.

——(2000) *Det kræver ledelse. Synspunkter om udvikling af den decentrale ledelse.*

——(2001) *Det gode lederskab. Redskaber til lederevaluering.* Copenhagen: Forlaget Kommuneinformation.

Personalestyrelsen/Finansministeriet [State Employer's Authority/Ministry of Finance] (2003) *Statens personale- og ledelsespolitik. Gør en forskel.*

Personalestyrelsen [State Employer's Authority] (2009) *Ny fleksibel masteruddannelse i offentlig ledelse. Formål, indhold og praktiske oplysninger.*

Index